FOUNDATIONS OF MEDICAL NEUROSCIENCE

Unraveling the Human Mind

Dr. Shrikant Akolekar

notionpress.com

INDIA • SINGAPORE • MALAYSIA

ISBN 979-8-90510-447-3

Contents

Preface

This E-Book was conceived with a single purpose: to make neuroscience accessible, integrated, and clinically meaningful for learners at every stage of their journey. Traditional textbooks often separate anatomy, physiology, and clinical application into isolated compartments. This work with integrated videos brings these domains together, showing how structure, function, and behavior form a continuous, interconnected whole.

The early chapters establish the essential architecture of the nervous system, its organization, vascular supply, and fundamental pathways. Subsequent sections explore the sensory, motor, limbic, and cognitive systems that give rise to perception, movement, memory, and thought. The final chapters extend these foundations into applied neuroscience, including neuropsychology, diagnostic reasoning, development, aging, and the neural basis of consciousness.

This integrated approach reflects the way the brain itself operates, not as a collection of isolated parts, but as a dynamic network whose components constantly interact. I hope that this e-book will help learners appreciate how the unity of concepts promotes a deeper understanding of both the science of the brain and the human experience it supports.

The E-Book format, combining text and multimedia, was chosen to enhance clarity, engagement, and retention. It is designed to be read linearly or explored modularly, depending on the learner's needs. Each chapter concludes with summary sheets, review questions, and clinical vignettes to reinforce key concepts and support exam preparation.

This book is the product of many years of teaching, writing, and reflection. It is offered with gratitude to the students who have shaped my teaching methodology of neuroscience and inspired me to share it with others.

Dr. Shrikant Akolekar
May 2026

Acknowledgments

This E-Book would not have been possible without the support and collaboration of many individuals. I am thankful to my wife, Manik, whose unwavering support has been the foundation of my academic journey. I extend heartfelt thanks to my students, past and present, whose curiosity, questions, and enthusiasm have shaped the structure and tone of this manuscript. Finally, I acknowledge the broader scientific community, researchers, clinicians, and educators whose collective efforts continue to expand our understanding of the nervous system. This book stands on the shoulders of their contributions.

I extend my heartfelt gratitude to Aishwarya, Jagadeeswar, Murali, and the consultants and staff of Notion Press, whose dedicated guidance and support were invaluable in bringing this manuscript to fruition.

Chapter 1

Introduction to the Central Nervous System

Click here to view
Chapter Video: https://youtu.be/nkwaO6ml__0

Overview of the Nervous System

The nervous system is the principal regulatory and communication network of the human body. It receives sensory information from the internal and external environment, integrates and interprets this input, and generates appropriate motor, autonomic, and behavioral responses. Traditionally, the nervous system is described in both structural and functional terms. Structurally, it is divided into the central nervous system (CNS), which includes the brain and spinal cord, and the peripheral nervous system (PNS), which comprises the cranial nerves, spinal nerves, and peripheral ganglia. Functionally, it is divided into the somatic nervous system, which mediates voluntary activities, and the autonomic nervous system (ANS), which regulates involuntary visceral functions. Although these divisions are useful for study, in practice, the nervous system functions as an integrated and highly coordinated unit.

Central Nervous System

The central nervous system consists of the brain and spinal cord, which are enclosed within the cranial cavity and vertebral canal, respectively. The CNS serves as the major integrative center of the body. It processes sensory input, generates motor output, and regulates higher mental functions such as memory, emotion, learning, and behavior. The brain is composed of the cerebral hemispheres, cerebellum, and brainstem. The brainstem, which includes the midbrain, pons, and medulla oblongata, is continuous inferiorly with the spinal cord at the foramen magnum. The CNS is protected by the skull, vertebral column, meninges, cerebrospinal fluid, and the blood-brain barrier, all of which preserve neural integrity and homeostasis.

Peripheral Nervous System

The peripheral nervous system includes 12 pairs of cranial nerves, 31 pairs of spinal nerves, and numerous peripheral ganglia. It forms the communication link between the CNS and the rest of the body. Sensory, or afferent, fibers transmit information from peripheral receptors to the CNS, whereas motor, or efferent, fibers convey impulses from the CNS to muscles, glands, and other target tissues. Through these pathways, the PNS enables both conscious sensation and coordinated motor activity.

Autonomic Nervous System

The autonomic nervous system is a specialized visceral motor system that regulates involuntary functions such as heart rate, blood pressure, respiration, digestion, and glandular secretion. It is divided into sympathetic and parasympathetic components, which often exert complementary or opposing effects on target organs. Autonomic pathways typically involve a two-neuron chain: a preganglionic neuron with its cell body in the CNS and a postganglionic neuron located in an autonomic ganglion. The hypothalamus is the principal central regulator of autonomic activity. It integrates visceral, endocrine, and emotional inputs and projects to autonomic nuclei in the brainstem and preganglionic neurons in the spinal cord.

Visceral afferent fibers accompany autonomic pathways and convey information from internal organs to the CNS. These fibers enter the spinal cord through the dorsal roots and ascend within general sensory pathways rather than through a distinct autonomic sensory tract.

Spinal Nerves

There are 31 pairs of spinal nerves: 8 cervical, 12 thoracic, 5 lumbar, 5 sacral, and 1 coccygeal. Each spinal nerve is formed by the union of a dorsal sensory root and a ventral motor root. The dorsal root ganglion contains the cell bodies of primary sensory neurons. Most spinal nerves exit the vertebral column through intervertebral foramina and contain mixed fibers, including somatic motor, somatic sensory, and autonomic components. This mixed composition enables spinal nerves to participate in sensory transmission, voluntary movement, and autonomic regulation.

Meninges

The central nervous system is enclosed by three protective connective tissue membranes: the dura mater, arachnoid mater, and pia mater. In the cranial cavity, the dura mater has two layers: an outer periosteal layer and an inner meningeal layer. In the spinal canal, only the meningeal layer persists as the spinal dura. The subarachnoid space, located between the arachnoid and pia mater, contains cerebrospinal fluid, which cushions and supports the CNS. The epidural and subdural spaces are normally potential spaces that become clinically significant in pathological conditions such as hemorrhage. Dural venous sinuses are located between the cranial dural layers and serve as major venous drainage channels. The tentorium cerebelli, a dural fold, separates the cerebellum from the occipital lobes.

Neurons: Structure and Functional Specialization

Neurons are the basic structural and functional units of the nervous system. They are highly specialized for the generation, conduction, and transmission of electrical impulses. A typical neuron consists of a cell body, or soma, which contains the nucleus and major organelles; dendrites, which receive incoming synaptic signals; an axon, which conducts action potentials away from the cell body; and synaptic terminals, which transmit signals to other neurons or effector cells. The axon hillock is the critical site where graded potentials are integrated and action potentials are initiated.

The neuronal cytoskeleton consists of microtubules, neurofilaments, and microfilaments. Microtubules are particularly important for axonal transport, which allows movement of proteins, organelles, and vesicles along the axon. Retrograde axonal transport is clinically significant because it can carry viruses and toxins, such as the rabies virus, from peripheral tissues to the CNS.

Nissl substance, which represents rough endoplasmic reticulum within the neuronal soma, is essential for protein synthesis. Loss of Nissl substance, known as chromatolysis, is a classic response to neuronal injury and reflects disruption of normal cellular metabolism.

Classification of Neurons

Neurons may be classified based on morphology, axonal length, and function. Morphologically, they are described as unipolar, bipolar, pseudounipolar, or multipolar. Based on axon length, neurons are classified as Golgi type I neurons with long axons, Golgi type II neurons with short axons, or anaxonic neurons that lack a distinct axon.

Functionally, neurons are categorized as sensory neurons, motor neurons, and interneurons. Sensory neurons transmit impulses from peripheral receptors to the CNS, motor neurons conduct impulses from the CNS to muscles and glands, and interneurons form complex integrative circuits entirely within the CNS. Interneurons constitute the majority of neurons in the CNS and are essential for reflexes, coordination, and higher cognitive functions.

Peripheral nerve fibers are also classified according to diameter, myelination, and conduction velocity using alphabetic and numeric systems. These classifications are important for understanding functional conduction properties and clinical nerve disorders.

Myelination and Nerve Conduction

Myelin is a lipid-rich insulating sheath that increases the speed and efficiency of impulse conduction. In the peripheral nervous system, myelin is produced by Schwann cells, whereas in the CNS it is formed by oligodendrocytes. Myelination begins in late fetal life and continues after birth, paralleling maturation of motor and sensory function. Conduction velocity increases with both axonal diameter and degree of myelination. Demyelinating disorders impair saltatory conduction and result in neurological deficits. A clinically important example is multiple sclerosis, a CNS demyelinating disease caused by immune-mediated injury to oligodendrocytes.

Neuroglia

Neuroglial cells are the most abundant supporting cells in the nervous system and are essential for maintaining the neural microenvironment. Unlike neurons, glial cells do not primarily conduct impulses, but they play indispensable roles in structural support, metabolic regulation, myelination, immune defence, and repair.

Astrocytes are the largest glial cells and are found in both Gray and white matter. They regulate extracellular ion balance, support the blood-brain barrier, and form glial scars after injury. Oligodendrocytes are responsible for the myelination of CNS axons and also provide metabolic support to neurons. Ependymal cells line the ventricles and central canal and contribute to cerebrospinal fluid production as part of the choroid plexus. Microglia are derived from mesodermal monocyte precursors and function as the resident macrophages of the CNS, migrating to sites of injury and phagocytosing cellular debris.

Together, neurons and neuroglia form the structural and functional foundation of the nervous system, allowing rapid communication, integration, and adaptive responses essential for survival.

Key Concepts

- CNS includes the brain and spinal cord; PNS includes cranial and spinal nerves.
- The somatic system is voluntary; the ANS is involuntary and uses twoneuron pathways.
- The hypothalamus is the highest autonomic control center.
- Spinal nerves are mixed nerves carrying somatic and autonomic fibers.
- Neurons are specialized for electrical conduction and classified by structure and function.
- Myelination increases conduction velocity; demyelination impairs function.
- Neuroglia support, protect, and maintain CNS homeostasis.

Review Questions

Q1. Which structure contains the cell bodies of primary sensory neurons
Answer: Dorsal root ganglion.

Q2. What is the major central regulator of autonomic output
Answer: Hypothalamus.

Q3. Which glial cell forms myelin in the CNS
Answer: Oligodendrocyte.

Q4. What is chromatolysis
Answer: Loss of Nissl substance following neuronal injury.

Q5. Which neuronal type is most abundant in the CNS
Answer: Interneurons.

References

1. Kandel ER et al. *Principles of Neural Science.* 5th ed. McGraw-Hill; 2013.
2. Nolte J. *The Human Brain.* 7th ed. Elsevier; 2016.
3. Purves D et al. *Neuroscience.* 6th ed. Oxford University Press; 2018.
4. Standring S. *Gray's Anatomy.* 42nd ed. Elsevier; 2020.

Chapter 2

Synaptic Communications

Click here to view
Chapter Video: https://youtu.be/tk0xphGendk

Synaptic Communication Overview

Synaptic communication is the fundamental mechanism by which neurons influence one another and coordinate nervous system activity. A synapse is a specialized junction through which the axon terminal of one neuron communicates with another neuron or an effector cell such as skeletal muscle. Depending on the site of contact, synapses may be classified as axodendritic, axosomatic, axoaxonic, or Dendrodendritic. Although their structural arrangements vary, all synapses serve the same essential purpose: The precise, modulated, and temporally regulated transfer of information.

Two major forms of synaptic transmission exist in the nervous system: chemical and electrical. Chemical synapses are the predominant type in the human central nervous system and allow highly adaptable signaling. Electrical synapses, although less common, provide rapid and synchronous communication in specialized neural circuits.

Chemical Synapses

Chemical synapses transmit signals by releasing neurotransmitters across a narrow synaptic cleft. This mode of transmission is characterized by the unidirectional flow of information from the presynaptic neuron to the postsynaptic cell. Unlike electrical synapses, chemical transmission involves a brief synaptic delay, usually around 0.5 milliseconds, but offers remarkable flexibility in regulating neural activity. Depending on the neurotransmitter released and the receptor activated, chemical synapses may exert excitatory, inhibitory, or modulatory effects.

Excitatory synaptic transmission typically produces an excitatory postsynaptic potential (EPSP), most commonly through sodium ion influx into the postsynaptic neuron. This depolarizes the membrane and increases the likelihood that the neuron will reach threshold and generate an action potential. Inhibitory transmission, in contrast, generates an inhibitory postsynaptic potential (IPSP), usually through chloride ion influx or potassium efflux. This hyperpolarizes the membrane and reduces the probability of neuronal firing.

Neurons receive thousands of synaptic inputs and integrate them continuously. Synaptic integration occurs through spatial summation, in which multiple synapses are activated simultaneously, and temporal summation, in which repeated impulses arrive in rapid succession from the same synapse. The final output of the neuron depends on the balance between excitatory and inhibitory influences.

Structure and Function of the Chemical Synapse

The presynaptic terminal contains synaptic vesicles filled with neurotransmitter, specialized active zones for vesicle docking, and voltage-gated calcium channels. When an action potential reaches the terminal, depolarization opens these calcium channels, allowing calcium ions to enter the presynaptic terminal. The influx of calcium is the critical trigger for vesicle fusion.

Synaptic vesicles then migrate to the presynaptic membrane and fuse with it through the action of SNARE proteins. This fusion results in exocytosis, releasing neurotransmitter molecules into the synaptic cleft. The neurotransmitter rapidly diffuses across the cleft and binds to receptors on the postsynaptic membrane.

Postsynaptic receptors are broadly classified into ionotropic and metabotropic types. Ionotropic receptors are ligand-gated ion channels that mediate rapid synaptic responses, often within milliseconds. Metabotropic receptors are G protein-coupled receptors that activate second messenger systems and produce slower but longer-lasting modulatory effects.

Termination of Neurotransmitter Action

For synaptic transmission to remain precise and efficient, neurotransmitter action must be terminated promptly after receptor activation. Several mechanisms contribute to this process. Reuptake into the presynaptic terminal is the major mechanism for monoamines such as serotonin, dopamine, and norepinephrine. Enzymatic degradation also plays an important role; for example, acetylcholinesterase rapidly breaks down acetylcholine in the synaptic cleft. In addition, some neurotransmitters diffuse away into the surrounding extracellular space.

These termination mechanisms are clinically significant because many pharmacologic agents act by altering neurotransmitter clearance, thereby modifying synaptic transmission.

Electrical Synapses

Electrical synapses are specialized junctions that allow direct electrical communication between adjacent cells. They are formed by gap junctions composed of connexons, with each connexon consisting of six connexin protein subunits. When connexons from adjacent cells align, they create a continuous intercellular channel that permits direct passage of ions and small signaling molecules.

This arrangement provides several important functional advantages. Electrical synapses allow bidirectional ionic flow, exhibit virtually no synaptic delay, support highly synchronized neuronal activity, and are resistant to synaptic fatigue. However, they offer less flexibility and modulation than chemical synapses.

In humans, electrical synapses are found in specialized locations such as the lateral vestibular nucleus, horizontal cells of the retina, and certain neuroglial networks, where rapid and coordinated signaling is essential.

Neurotransmitters and Receptors

Neurotransmitters are chemical messengers that mediate synaptic transmission. Glutamate is the principal excitatory neurotransmitter in the central nervous system and acts primarily through NMDA, AMPA, and Kainate receptors. Excess glutamate release contributes to excitotoxic neuronal injury, particularly in ischemic stroke.

Gamma-aminobutyric acid (GABA) is the major inhibitory neurotransmitter in the brain. It acts through GABA_A receptors, which are ionotropic chloride channels, and metabotropic GABA_B receptors. Benzodiazepines enhance GABA_A receptor activity and are widely used as anxiolytic and anticonvulsant agents.

Glycine is an important inhibitory neurotransmitter in the spinal cord and brainstem. Its receptors are chloride-permeable ion channels, and blockade by toxins such as strychnine can result in severe muscle spasms.

Acetylcholine is essential for neuromuscular transmission, autonomic signaling, and cognition. It acts through both nicotinic and muscarinic receptors. Degeneration of cholinergic neurons in the basal forebrain is associated with cognitive decline in Alzheimer's disease.

Monoamine neurotransmitters also play key roles in CNS function. Dopamine, produced in the substantia nigra and ventral tegmental area, regulates movement, motivation, and reward. Degeneration of dopaminergic neurons in the substantia nigra is a hallmark of Parkinson's disease. Norepinephrine, primarily from the locus coeruleus, supports arousal and attention. Serotonin, produced in the raphe nuclei, modulates mood, sleep, and affective behavior. Histamine, synthesized in the tuberomammillary nucleus, promotes wakefulness and alertness.

Ionotropic and Metabotropic Receptors

Ionotropic receptors mediate fast synaptic transmission by directly opening ion channels upon neurotransmitter binding. Examples include NMDA and AMPA glutamate receptors, GABA_A receptors, and nicotinic acetylcholine receptors. Their effects are rapid and short-lived.

Metabotropic receptors act indirectly through G proteins and second messenger systems. Although slower in onset, they produce longer lasting and more diverse modulatory effects. Examples include muscarinic acetylcholine receptors, GABA_B receptors, and most monoamine receptors. These receptors are major targets for many neurologic and psychiatric drugs.

Synaptic Pharmacology and Clinical Correlations

Synaptic transmission is highly susceptible to pharmacologic modulation. Drugs may alter neurotransmitter synthesis, vesicular storage, release, receptor binding, reuptake, or degradation. For example, alpha-methyltyrosine inhibits catecholamine synthesis, whereas reserpine depletes monoamines by blocking vesicular storage.

Botulinum toxin causes flaccid paralysis by cleaving SNARE proteins and preventing acetylcholine release at the neuromuscular junction. In contrast, tetanus toxin cleaves synaptobrevin in inhibitory interneurons, blocking the release of GABA and glycine and producing spastic paralysis, trismus, and opisthotonus.

Neuropsychiatric drugs also exert their effects at synapses. Benzodiazepines enhance GABA_A receptor activity, producing anxiolytic and anticonvulsant effects. Selective serotonin reuptake inhibitors (SSRIs) increase synaptic serotonin levels by blocking reuptake. Cocaine inhibits the reuptake of dopamine, norepinephrine, and serotonin, resulting in euphoria and sympathetic stimulation.

NMDA Receptor Physiology and Synaptic Plasticity

The NMDA receptor is a specialized glutamate receptor with unique properties important for synaptic plasticity and learning. At resting membrane potential, the receptor channel is blocked by magnesium ions. Activation requires both glutamate binding and sufficient postsynaptic depolarization to displace the magnesium block. Once activated, the receptor allows calcium influx, which initiates intracellular signaling pathways involved in long-term potentiation (LTP), a key cellular mechanism underlying learning and memory.

Neuromuscular Junction

The neuromuscular junction is a highly specialized cholinergic synapse between a motor neuron and skeletal muscle. When acetylcholine is released from the motor nerve terminal, it binds to nicotinic receptors on the muscle end plate, causing sodium influx and depolarization that triggers muscle contraction.

This process can be altered pharmacologically. Curare acts as a competitive antagonist at nicotinic receptors and causes paralysis. Organophosphate compounds inhibit acetylcholinesterase, leading to excessive accumulation of acetylcholine, persistent depolarization, and depolarization block.

Together, chemical and electrical synapses form the basis of neural communication, enabling rapid signal transmission, complex integration, plasticity, and pharmacologic modulation across the nervous system.

High-Yield Summary

- Synapses are **chemical or electrical**
- EPSP = depolarization; IPSP = hyperpolarization
- Synaptic integration via **spatial + temporal summation**

- Ionotropic = fast; metabotropic = modulatory
- Neurotransmitter removal: **reuptake, degradation, diffusion**
- NMDA receptors require **dual activation**
- Tetanus vs botulinum toxins → opposite effects

USMLE Pearls

- **Botulinum toxin → flaccid paralysis (↓ ACh)**
- **Tetanus toxin → spastic paralysis (↓ GABA/glycine)**
- **SSRIs increase synaptic serotonin via reuptake inhibition**
- **NMDA receptors act as coincidence detectors**
- **Cocaine increases monoamines → sympathetic activation**

Key Concepts

- Synapses transmit information through chemical or electrical mechanisms.
- Chemical synapses allow excitatory, inhibitory, and modulatory signaling.
- EPSPs and IPSPs undergo spatial and temporal summation.
- Ionotropic receptors mediate fast responses; metabotropic receptors mediate slow modulation.
- Neurotransmitter action is terminated by reuptake, degradation, or diffusion.
- Pharmacologic agents target synthesis, release, reuptake, degradation, and receptor activity.
- NMDA receptors require both ligand binding and depolarization, enabling LTP.
- Tetanus and botulinum toxins illustrate contrasting effects on synaptic transmission.

Review Questions

Q1. What ion movement typically generates an EPSP?
Answer: Sodium influx.

Q2. Which receptor type mediates fast synaptic transmission?
Answer: Ionotropic receptors.

Q3. What is the mechanism of botulinum toxin?
Answer: Cleavage of SNARE proteins, preventing ACh release.

Q4. Which neurotransmitter is the major inhibitory transmitter in the spinal cord?
Answer: Glycine.

Q5. Why are NMDA receptors important for synaptic plasticity?
Answer: They require both glutamate binding and depolarization, enabling long-term potentiation.

References

1. Kandel ER et al. *Principles of Neural Science.* 5th ed. McGraw-Hill; 2013.
2. Purves D et al. *Neuroscience.* 6th ed. Oxford University Press; 2018.
3. Bear MF, Connors BW, Paradiso MA. *Neuroscience: Exploring the Brain.* 4th ed. Wolters Kluwer; 2015.
4. Blumenfeld H. *Neuroanatomy Through Clinical Cases.* 3rd ed. Sinauer Associates; 2021.

Chapter 3

Cellular Organization (Neurocytology)

Click here to view
Chapter Video: https://youtu.be/SVmvAKj2-1A

The early neural tube is lined by a rapidly proliferating population of neuroepithelial cells, forming a pseudostratified columnar neuroepithelium. These cells undergo repeated mitotic cycles, generating a proliferative (ventricular) zone that serves as the source of all intrinsic neural elements of the central nervous system. As development progresses, successive waves of proliferation give rise to the major cellular constituents of the CNS.

Formation of the Mantle and Marginal Layers

The first wave of neuroepithelial proliferation produces neuroblasts, which migrate outward to form the mantle layer, the future grey matter of the spinal cord and brainstem. Neuroblasts extend axonal processes peripherally, establishing the marginal layer, which becomes white matter as these axons myelinate.

A second wave of proliferation produces glioblasts, which are precursors to astrocytes and oligodendrocytes. After neurogenesis and gliogenesis are completed, the original neuroepithelial layer develops into the ependymal layer, which remains in adults as the lining of the ventricular system.

In contrast to these intrinsic CNS derivatives, microglia arise from mesodermal bone marrow precursors. They migrate into the CNS during development and function as resident macrophages, participating in immune surveillance and phagocytosis.

Thus, from inside outward, the neural tube differentiates into three fundamental layers:

1. Ependymal layer
2. Mantle layer (future grey matter)
3. Marginal layer (future white matter)

Dorsoventral Patterning: Alar and Basal Plates

By the fourth week, a shallow longitudinal groove, the sulcus limitans, appears on the inner surface of the neural tube. This groove divides the mantle layer into:

- Dorsal alar plate → sensory (afferent) regions
- Ventral basal plate → motor (efferent) regions

These plates are connected dorsally by the roof plate and ventrally by the floor plate, both of which serve as signaling centers guiding neuronal differentiation. **Functional Columns of the Spinal Cord. The alar and basal plates give rise to distinct functional columns:**

Plate	Column	Distribution	Function
Alar (sensory)	General Somatic Afferent (GSA)	Entire spinal cord	Sensation from the skin, muscle, and joints
	General Visceral Afferent (GVA)	Thoracolumbar & sacral regions	Sensation from viscera, vessels
Basal (motor)	General Somatic Efferent (GSE)	Entire spinal cord	Motor to skeletal muscle
	General Visceral Efferent (GVE)	Thoracolumbar & sacral regions	Preganglionic autonomic fibers

Neuroblasts in the basal plate extend axons outward to form motor roots, while neural crest–derived cells in the dorsal root ganglia send central processes into the alar plate and peripheral processes to sensory receptors. This establishes the fundamental afferent–efferent organization of the spinal cord.

Myelination and Fiber Types

Myelination begins relatively late in development—during the third trimester, and continues well into the postnatal period, reflecting the prolonged maturation of neural circuits. Myelin is produced by:

- Oligodendrocytes in the CNS
- Schwann cells in the PNS

These glial cells wrap their plasma membranes around axons in concentric layers, forming a multilamellar sheath that enables saltatory conduction and dramatically increases conduction velocity.

Myelinated Vs. Unmyelinated Fibers

Fiber Type	Myelination	Conduction Speed	Function
Aalpha, Abeta	Heavily myelinated	Fastest	Proprioception, touch
Adelta, B fibers	Lightly myelinated	Intermediate	Pain (fast), autonomic preganglionic
C fibers	Unmyelinated	Slowest	Pain (slow), temperature, autonomic postganglionic

C fibers, though ensheathed by Schwann cells, lack true myelin wrapping and conduct impulses slowly.

Postnatal Maturation, Cellular Lineages, and Molecular Patterning.

Neuroblasts, the terminally differentiated precursors of neurons, complete their final mitotic divisions during embryogenesis and early fetal life. Once neurons are generated and migrate to their definitive locations, they permanently exit the cell cycle. As a result, neuronal regeneration in the mature CNS is extremely limited, a principle with profound clinical implications. In contrast, neuroglial cells retain proliferative capacity throughout life, enabling them to participate in tissue maintenance, metabolic support, immune surveillance, and repair.

Postnatal maturation of the nervous system is an extended process. Although the majority of neurons are present at birth, the CNS continues to undergo axonal elongation, dendritic arborization, synaptic refinement, and progressive myelination well into childhood and adolescence. These processes underlie the acquisition of motor coordination, cognitive development, and higher-order neural functions.

Neurocytological Derivatives and Tumorigenesis

The embryonic origins of neural cells are reflected in their associated pathologies.

- Neuroblastoma, arising from primitive sympathetic neuroblasts, accounts for 7–10% of pediatric malignancies. Despite its embryonic derivation, neuroblastoma often demonstrates a favorable prognosis in younger children due to its capacity for spontaneous regression or differentiation.
- Glioblastoma, in contrast, arises from malignant transformation of glioblasts or their mature derivatives. It is a highly aggressive astrocytic tumor that predominantly affects adults and carries a poor prognosis despite multimodal therapy.

These contrasting neoplasms underscore the divergent biological behaviors of neuronal and glial lineages.

Molecular Patterning of the Neural Tube

The growth, regional specification, and differentiation of the neural tube are governed by a precisely orchestrated interplay of signaling molecules and transcriptional regulators. These molecular gradients establish positional identity along both the anterior–posterior and dorsal–ventral axes.

Anterior–Posterior Patterning

Development of the rostral neural tube, which gives rise to the brain, is initiated by the expression of homeobox (HOX) genes and related transcription factors. These genes encode positional information that determines the identity of forebrain, midbrain, and hindbrain regions.

Dorsal–Ventral Patterning

Dorsoventral patterning is established by opposing gradients of Sonic hedgehog (Shh) and bone morphogenetic proteins (BMPs):

- Sonic hedgehog (Shh)
    - Secreted by the notochord and floor plate
    - Induces differentiation of ventral motor neurons
    - Establishes the basal plate (motor domain)

- Bone morphogenetic proteins (BMPs)
    - Secreted by the overlying ectoderm and roof plate
    - Promote differentiation of dorsal sensory interneurons
    - Establish the alar plate (sensory domain)

This molecular antagonism creates sharply defined sensory and motor territories within the developing spinal cord and brainstem.

Functional Organization of the Spinal Cord (Integrated Review)

The dorsoventral patterning of the neural tube gives rise to the major functional columns of the spinal cord:

Sensory (Afferent) Columns Alar Plate

Column	Distribution	Function
General Somatic Afferent (GSA)	Entire spinal cord	Sensation from the skin, muscle, and joints
General Visceral Afferent (GVA)	Thoracolumbar & sacral regions	Sensation from the viscera and blood vessels

Motor (Efferent) Columns Basal Plate

Column	Distribution	Function
General Somatic Efferent (GSE)	Entire spinal cord	Motor innervation to skeletal muscle
General Visceral Efferent (GVE)	Thoracolumbar & sacral regions	Preganglionic autonomic fibers

The dorsal root ganglia, derived from neural crest cells, extend central processes into the alar plate and peripheral processes to sensory receptors, completing the afferent limb of spinal circuitry. Motor neurons in the basal plate extend axons outward to form the ventral roots.

Myelination and Fiber Classification (Integrated Review)

Myelination begins in the third trimester and continues into adolescence. Oligodendrocytes in the CNS and Schwann cells in the PNS wrap axons in concentric layers of membrane, forming the myelin sheath that enables saltatory conduction.

Myelinated and Unmyelinated Fibers

Fiber Type	Myelination	Conduction Velocity	Functional Role
Aalpha, Abeta	Heavily myelinated	Fastest	Proprioception, fine touch
Adelta, B-fibers	Lightly myelinated	Intermediate	Fast pain, autonomic preganglionic
C fibers	Unmyelinated	Slowest	Slow pain, temperature, and autonomic postganglionic

C fibers are ensheathed by Schwann cells but lack true myelin spiraling, accounting for their slow conduction.

Review questions

Q1. A mutation in Sonic hedgehog signaling would most directly impair the development of which neural structure?
Answer: Ventral motor neurons (basal plate).

Q2. A newborn with absent deep tendon reflexes is found to have agenesis of the basal plate. Which functional column is missing?
Answer: General somatic efferent (GSE).

Q3. A tumor arising from primitive sympathetic neuroblasts is most likely to present in which age group?
Answer: Infants and young children (neuroblastoma).

Q4. Which glial cell type is derived from mesoderm rather than neuroectoderm?
Answer: Microglia.

Q5. A lesion affecting the alar plate during development would impair which function?
Answer: Sensory processing (GSA and GVA).

Q6. A child presents with sharp, well-localized pain followed by a dull ache. Which fiber types mediate these sensations?
Answer: Sharp pain → Adelta fibers ; Dull pain → C fibers

Q7. Which CNS layer persists into adulthood as the ependymal lining of the ventricles?
Answer: The ventricular (neuroepithelial) layer.

Q8. A mutation in BMP signaling would most directly affect which neural derivatives?
Answer: Dorsal sensory interneurons (alar plate).

Q9. Which of the following best explains why CNS neurons do not regenerate effectively?
Answer: Neuroblasts become post-mitotic and permanently exit the cell cycle.

Q10. A 60-year-old patient presents with a rapidly progressive brain tumor showing pseudopalisading necrosis. Which embryologic precursor cell type is implicated?
Answer: Glioblast (astrocytic lineage).

Clinical vignette

Vignette 1 - Shh Signaling Defect
A newborn presents with midline facial defects and holoprosencephaly.
Concept: Impaired Shh signaling disrupts ventral neural tube patterning and forebrain separation.

Vignette 2 - Neuroblastoma
A 2-year-old child presents with an abdominal mass and elevated catecholamine metabolites.
Diagnosis: Neuroblastoma
Concept: Tumor of sympathetic neuroblasts; often has a favorable prognosis in infants.

Vignette 3 - Glioblastoma
A 58-year-old man develops rapidly progressive neurological deficits. MRI shows a ring-enhancing lesion with central necrosis.
Diagnosis: Glioblastoma multiforme
Concept: Malignant transformation of glioblastoma lineage; highly aggressive.

Vignette 4 - Dorsal–Ventral Patterning
A mutation in BMP signaling impairs the development of dorsal spinal cord structures.
Expected deficit: Loss of sensory interneurons derived from the alar plate.

Vignette 5 - (Dorsal Root Ganglion Development)
A newborn exhibits absent pain and temperature sensation in a dermatomal distribution. Biopsy reveals the absence of neurons in the dorsal root ganglion.
Concept: DRG neurons arise from neural crest; failure of migration → sensory deficits.

Vignette 6- Myelination Disorders
A 3-year-old child presents with delayed motor milestones and hypotonia. MRI shows diffuse hypomyelination.
Diagnosis: Leukodystrophy
Concept: Oligodendrocyte dysfunction impairs CNS myelination.

References

1. Snell's Clinical Neuroanatomy
Snell RS. *Clinical Neuroanatomy*. 8th ed. Wolters Kluwer.

2. Gray's Anatomy for Students
Drake RL, Vogl W, Mitchell AWM. *Gray's Anatomy for Students*. 4th ed. Elsevier.

3. Neuroanatomy Through Clinical Cases
Blumenfeld H. *Neuroanatomy Through Clinical Cases*. 3rd ed. Sinauer Associates.

Chapter 4
Autonomic Nervous System

Click here to view
Chapter Video: https://youtu.be/l8R0OIRmx0A

Introduction

The autonomic nervous system (ANS) is the principal visceral motor system of the body. It regulates the internal environment by controlling the activity of smooth muscle, cardiac muscle, and glands, thereby maintaining homeostasis. Unlike the somatic nervous system, which mediates voluntary control of skeletal muscle, the autonomic nervous system functions largely outside conscious awareness. Through the continuous adjustments in organ function, it helps maintain cardiovascular stability, thermoregulation, digestion, respiration, and visceral reflexes.

The ANS operates in close association with visceral afferent pathways, local reflex arcs, and higher central regulatory centers. Its organization is hierarchical, with the hypothalamus serving as the highest integrative center for autonomic function.

Somatic and Autonomic Nervous Systems: Functional Comparison

The somatic nervous system is primarily responsible for voluntary movement and conscious sensory-motor control. It uses a single lower motor neuron that extends directly from the central nervous system to skeletal muscle. This system enables precise and rapid control of movement.

In contrast, the autonomic nervous system regulates involuntary visceral activity. Its efferent pathway typically consists of a two-neuron chain: a preganglionic neuron located in the central nervous system and a postganglionic neuron located in a peripheral autonomic ganglion. The ANS supplies smooth muscle, cardiac muscle, glands, and visceral organs. Its primary function is to maintain internal physiological balance and adapt organ activity to changing demands.

Although autonomic outflow is mediated by a two-neuron peripheral pathway, overall autonomic control follows a broader three-level hierarchy involving hypothalamic centers, brainstem and spinal cord preganglionic neurons, and peripheral ganglia.

Divisions of the Autonomic Nervous System

The autonomic nervous system consists of two major divisions: the sympathetic nervous system and the parasympathetic nervous system. These systems usually exert complementary or opposing effects on target organs, allowing fine regulation of visceral function.

The sympathetic division is classically associated with the "fight or flight" response and prepares the body for stress, exercise, and emergencies. The parasympathetic division is associated with "rest and digest" functions and promotes energy conservation, digestion, and restorative processes.

Sympathetic Nervous System (Origin and Organization)

The sympathetic nervous system has a thoracolumbar outflow. Preganglionic sympathetic neurons are in the intermediolateral cell column, or lateral horn, of the spinal cord from T1 to L2 spinal segments. Their axons exit the spinal cord through the anterior roots, enter the spinal nerves, and pass through the white rami communicantes to reach the sympathetic trunk.

Once within the sympathetic chain, preganglionic fibers may follow several pathways. They may synapse in a ganglion at the same spinal level, ascend to cervical ganglia, descend to lumbar or sacral ganglia, or pass through the chain without synapsing to form thoracic splanchnic nerves that relay in prevertebral ganglia.

Postganglionic Pathways

Postganglionic sympathetic fibers distributed through the Gray rami communicantes rejoin spinal nerves and supply the body wall and limbs. These fibers mediate vasomotor control of blood vessels, sudomotor innervation of sweat glands, and pilomotor innervation of arrector pili muscles.

Fibers arising from the superior cervical ganglion form plexuses around the carotid arteries. The internal carotid plexus supplies cranial structures, including the dilator pupillae muscle, superior tarsal muscle, mucosal glands, lacrimal gland, and intracranial blood vessels. The external carotid plexus supplies sympathetic fibers to structures of the face and scalp.

Sympathetic cardiopulmonary nerves arise primarily from upper thoracic ganglia and supply the heart, trachea, and bronchi. These fibers increase heart rate, enhance myocardial contractility, and promote bronchodilation.

Preganglionic fibers that pass through the sympathetic chain without synapsing form thoracic splanchnic nerves, including the greater, lesser, and least splanchnic nerves. These fibers synapse in prevertebral ganglia such as the celiac, superior mesenteric, and aorticorenal ganglia, from which postganglionic fibers supply abdominal and pelvic viscera.

Neurotransmitters

Sympathetic preganglionic neurons release acetylcholine, which acts on nicotinic receptors in autonomic ganglia. Most sympathetic postganglionic neurons release norepinephrine, which acts on adrenergic receptors at target organs. An important exception is the sympathetic innervation of sweat glands, where postganglionic fibers are cholinergic and release acetylcholine.

Parasympathetic Nervous System (Origin and Organization)

The parasympathetic nervous system has a craniosacral outflow. Preganglionic neurons arise from specific nuclei in the brainstem and from sacral spinal cord segments S2 to S4.

The cranial parasympathetic outflow is carried by cranial nerves III, VII, IX, and X. The sacral outflow reaches pelvic organs through pelvic splanchnic nerves.

Cranial Parasympathetic Ganglia and Targets

Parasympathetic fibers associated with the oculomotor nerve synapse in the ciliary ganglion and supply the sphincter pupillae and ciliary muscle, mediating pupillary constriction and accommodation.

Fibers carried by the facial nerve synapse in the pterygopalatine ganglion to supply the lacrimal, nasal, and palatine glands, and in the submandibular ganglion to supply the submandibular and sublingual salivary glands.

Glossopharyngeal nerve fibers synapse in the Otic ganglion and provide secretomotor innervation to the parotid gland.

The vagus nerve provides extensive parasympathetic innervation to thoracic and abdominal viscera through intramural ganglia located within or near the walls of target organs. It regulates cardiac slowing, bronchoconstriction, gastrointestinal motility, and glandular secretion.

Sacral Parasympathetic System

Parasympathetic fibers from S2 to S4 supply the distal colon, rectum, urinary bladder, and reproductive organs. These fibers are essential for micturition, defecation, and sexual function.

Neurotransmitters

Parasympathetic preganglionic neurons release acetylcholine, which acts on nicotinic receptors in autonomic ganglia. Postganglionic parasympathetic neurons also release acetylcholine, which acts on muscarinic receptors at target organs.

Muscarinic receptor subtypes mediate varied effects. M1, M3, and M5 receptors are generally excitatory and promote glandular secretion and smooth muscle contraction. M2 and M4 receptors are generally inhibitory and play important roles in slowing heart rate and modulating neural activity.

Enteric Nervous System

The enteric nervous system is a highly specialized intrinsic neural network located within the wall of the gastrointestinal tract. It is often referred to as the "little brain" of the gut because of its capacity for autonomous reflex activity. The enteric nervous system consists primarily of two interconnected plexuses. The myenteric (Auerbach) plexus, located between the circular and longitudinal muscle layers, regulates gastrointestinal motility and peristalsis. The submucosal (Meissner) plexus, located in the submucosa, regulates glandular secretion, local blood flow, and absorption.

Although the enteric nervous system is influenced by sympathetic and parasympathetic input, it is capable of functioning independently through local reflex circuits. This intrinsic autonomy is essential for coordinated digestion and normal gastrointestinal function. Together, the sympathetic, parasympathetic, and enteric divisions of the autonomic nervous system maintain internal physiological stability and enable rapid adaptation to both internal and external changes.

Key Concepts

- ANS is involuntary and regulates smooth muscle, cardiac muscle, and glands.
- The somatic system uses a single neuron; the ANS uses a two-neuron chain.
- Sympathetic outflow is thoracolumbar (T1–L2); parasympathetic is craniosacral.
- The sympathetic chain allows fibers to ascend, descend, or pass through as splanchnic nerves.
- Parasympathetic ganglia are located near or within target organs.
- Sympathetic postganglionic fibers are mostly noradrenergic; parasympathetic are cholinergic.
- ENS operates independently but is modulated by ANS inputs.

Review Questions

Q1. Where are sympathetic preganglionic neurons located
Answer: Lateral horn of spinal cord segments T1–L2.

Q2. Which ganglion receives parasympathetic fibers from the oculomotor nerve
Answer: Ciliary ganglion.

Q3. What neurotransmitter is released by most sympathetic postganglionic neurons
Answer: Noradrenaline.

Q4. Which plexus of the enteric nervous system regulates peristalsis
Answer: Myenteric (Auerbach's) plexus.

Q5. Which cranial nerve carries the majority of parasympathetic outflow to thoracic and abdominal organs
Answer: Vagus nerve (CN X).

References

1. Kandel ER et al. *Principles of Neural Science.* 5th ed. McGrawHill; 2013.
2. Standring S. *Gray's Anatomy.* 42nd ed. Elsevier; 2020.
3. Barrett KE et al. *Ganong's Review of Medical Physiology.* 26th ed. McGrawHill; 2019.
4. Purves D et al. *Neuroscience.* 6th ed. Oxford University Press; 2018.

Chapter 5

Cerebrum: External Features

Click here to view
Chapter Video: https://youtu.be/hYNa75bSwQo

Overview of the Cerebrum

The cerebrum is the largest and most functionally complex component of the central nervous system. Together with the cerebellum and brainstem, it forms the triad of major brain divisions, yet the cerebrum alone contains nearly 85% of all neurons. Every sensory modality, motor function, cognitive process, emotional state, and memory system is represented somewhere within its extensive neural architecture.

Although the two cerebral hemispheres share a mirrored structural plan, certain functions are preferentially processed in one hemisphere—a phenomenon known as lateralization or hemispheric dominance. Language, for example, is typically dominant in the left hemisphere, while visuospatial processing is more prominent in the right.

Interhemispheric Separation and Connectivity

The right and left hemispheres are separated by the deep interhemispheric (longitudinal) fissure, yet remain intimately connected by the corpus callosum, the largest commissural fiber bundle in the brain. When the superior portions of the hemispheres are removed during anatomical dissection, the corpus callosum appears as a broad, arched structure forming the floor of the fissure.

This commissural system enables:

- Integration of sensory information
- Coordination of bilateral motor activity
- Unification of cognitive and emotional processes

The corpus callosum is essential for interhemispheric communication and functional coherence.

Cerebral Cortex and Subcortical White Matter

A coronal section through the cerebrum reveals the cerebral cortex, a thin but highly convoluted sheet of grey matter composed of layered neuronal cell bodies. The surface is thrown into:

- Gyri — elevated folds
- Sulci — intervening grooves

This pattern of convolutions dramatically increases cortical surface area, supporting the enormous computational capacity of the human brain.

Beneath the cortex lies the subcortical white matter, composed of myelinated axons organized into three major fiber systems:

- Association fibers — interconnect regions within the same hemisphere
- Commissural fibers — link corresponding areas of the two hemispheres
- Projection fibers — connect the cortex with the brainstem, spinal cord, and subcortical nuclei

Embedded within this white matter are deep grey matter structures, including the thalamus, basal nuclei, and amygdaloid complex, which participate in sensory relay, motor modulation, emotional processing, and memory formation.

External Morphology of the Cerebral Hemispheres

Each cerebral hemisphere is described in terms of:

- Three poles
  - Frontal pole
  - Temporal pole
  - Occipital pole
- Three surfaces
  - Superolateral surface
  - Medial surface
  - Inferior surface
- Three borders
  - Superomedial border

- Inferomedial border
- Inferolateral border

The superomedial border separates the superolateral and medial surfaces, while the inferolateral border demarcates the superolateral and inferior surfaces. The inferomedial border curves around the cerebral peduncle and is formed by the medial aspect of the uncus and parahippocampal gyrus.

Lobar Organization of the Cerebrum

The cerebrum is divided into four major lobes—frontal, parietal, temporal, and occipital—named for the cranial bones that overlie them. A combination of major sulci and imaginary lines defines these lobes.

Key landmarks include:

- Central sulcus — separates frontal and parietal lobes
- Lateral sulcus (Sylvian fissure) — separates the temporal lobe from the frontal and parietal lobes
- Parietooccipital sulcus — separates parietal and occipital lobes (primarily on the medial surface)
- Preoccipital notch — helps define the anterior boundary of the occipital lobe

These boundaries provide the framework for understanding cortical topography and functional localization.

Major Sulci, Lobar Boundaries, and Surface Anatomy

The external anatomy of the cerebrum is defined by a series of prominent sulci and fissures that demarcate the major lobes and guide the organization of cortical functions.

Central Sulcus

The central sulcus is the most striking landmark on the superolateral surface.

- Begins near the superomedial border
- Descends obliquely downward and forward
- Terminates just above the lateral sulcus

It separates the frontal lobe (anterior) from the parietal lobe (posterior) and demarcates the primary motor cortex (precentral gyrus) from the primary somatosensory cortex (postcentral gyrus).

Lateral Sulcus (Sylvian Fissure)

The lateral sulcus originates on the inferior surface of the forebrain.

- Its short stem ascends onto the superolateral surface
- Divides into three rami:
    - Horizontal ramus
    - Ascending ramus
    - Posterior ramus (longest)

This sulcus separates the temporal lobe below from the frontal and parietal lobes above.

ParietoOccipital Sulcus

Located primarily on the medial surface, this deep vertical groove separates the parietal and occipital lobes.

Its upper end curves slightly onto the superolateral surface, serving as a key landmark for defining the posterior extent of the parietal lobe.

Preoccipital Notch and Imaginary Boundaries

Because the occipital lobe lacks sharply defined external boundaries, anatomists rely on an imaginary line drawn between:

- The preoccipital notch (inferolateral border)
- The upturned end of the parieto-occipital sulcus

This line marks the anterior limit of the occipital lobe.
Using these boundaries:

- Region between the central sulcus and this line → parietal lobe
- Area anterior to the central sulcus and above the lateral sulcus → frontal lobe
- Region below the lateral sulcus → temporal lobe

Detailed Surface Anatomy of the Lobes

Frontal Lobe

The frontal lobe occupies the anterior one-third of the hemisphere.

Key Sulci and Gyri

- Precentral sulcus — anterior to the central sulcus; defines the precentral gyrus
- Superior, middle, and inferior frontal gyri — formed by horizontally oriented sulci
- Prefrontal cortex — anterior region associated with executive function, judgment, and personality

Inferior Frontal Gyrus

Subdivided by the horizontal and ascending rami of the lateral sulcus into:

- Pars orbitalis
- Pars triangularis
- Pars opercularis

The pars opercularis + pars triangularis form Broca's area in the dominant hemisphere.

Orbitofrontal Surface

- Gyrus rectus along the inferomedial border
- Olfactory sulcus lateral to it, housing the olfactory tract and bulb
- Several irregular orbital gyri laterally

Insula

Deep within the lateral sulcus lies the insula, a concealed cortical region covered by the opercula of the frontal, parietal, and temporal lobes.

Separated by the circular sulcus, the insula participates in:

- Visceral sensation
- Autonomic integration
- Emotional processing
- Interoceptive awareness

Parietal Lobe

The parietal lobe has less sharply defined boundaries.

Boundaries
- Anterior: central sulcus
- Posterior: line from parieto-occipital sulcus to preoccipital notch
- Inferior: line extending backward from the posterior ramus of the lateral sulcus

Key Structures
- Postcentral gyrus — primary somatosensory cortex
- Postcentral sulcus — posterior boundary of postcentral gyrus
- Intraparietal sulcus — divides the parietal lobe into:
  - Superior parietal lobule
  - Inferior parietal lobule

The inferior parietal lobule contains:
- Supramarginal gyrus
- Angular gyrus

Both are critical for language, spatial awareness, and multimodal integration.

Temporal Lobe: Superolateral and Inferior Surfaces

The temporal lobe occupies the region beneath the inferolateral border of the cerebral hemisphere and is bounded superiorly by the lateral sulcus and its posterior ramus. On the superolateral surface, two prominent sulci—the superior temporal sulcus and inferior temporal sulcus—divide the lobe into:
- Superior temporal gyrus — primary auditory cortex and auditory association areas
- Middle temporal gyrus — multimodal integration, semantic processing
- Inferior temporal gyrus — high-order visual processing, object recognition

These gyri support auditory perception, language comprehension, and complex visual analysis.

Inferior Surface of the Temporal Lobe

When viewed from below, two long, parallel sulci become evident:

- Occipitotemporal sulcus — lateral
- Collateral sulcus — medial, deeper

Between them lies the occipitotemporal gyrus, a region essential for:

- Face recognition (fusiform face area)
- Object identification
- High-order visual association

This gyrus plays a central role in visual categorization and recognition memory.

Parahippocampal Gyrus and Uncus

Medial to the collateral sulcus lies the parahippocampal gyrus, a major component of the limbic system. It curves medially and posteriorly to form the uncus, a hookshaped structure overlying:

- The amygdala
- The anterior hippocampus

The uncus is clinically significant because:

- Uncal herniation compresses the oculomotor nerve
- It is a key site for olfactory and emotional processing

Posteriorly, the parahippocampal gyrus narrows into the isthmus, which connects it to the cingulate gyrus, forming part of the limbic ring.

Cingulate Gyrus and Medial Limbic Cortex

The cingulate gyrus arches over the corpus callosum, following its curvature.

The cingulate sulcus runs parallel to it, separating limbic cortex from the medial frontal and parietal lobes.

Functions of the cingulate region include:

- Emotional regulation
- Motivational behavior
- Autonomic integration
- Cognitive control

This region forms the dorsal limbic belt, linking emotion with executive function.

Medial Surface of the Occipital Lobe

Two major fissures dominate the medial occipital surface:

ParietoOccipital Sulcus

- Deep vertical groove
- Separates parietal and occipital lobes

Calcarine Sulcus

- Extends posteriorly from the occipital pole
- Joins the parieto-occipital sulcus at an acute angle
- Contains the stria of Gennari, a band of white fibers characteristic of the primary visual cortex (striate cortex)

This region corresponds to Brodmann area 17, the site of initial cortical visual processing.

Cuneus and Lingual Gyrus

The medial occipital lobe contains two important gyri:

- Cuneus — triangular wedge between the parieto-occipital and calcarine sulci; processes the inferior visual field
- Lingual gyrus — inferior to the calcarine sulcus; participates in visual association, including pattern and word recognition

Together, these structures form the cortical foundation for visual perception and interpretation.

Limbic System Surface Anatomy

The medial aspect of the hemisphere contains a ring of interconnected cortical and subcortical structures forming the limbic system, responsible for emotion, memory, motivation, and autonomic regulation.

Surface components include:

- Cingulate gyrus
- Subcallosal area
- Isthmus of the cingulate gyrus
- Parahippocampal gyrus

- Uncus
- Amygdala (deep to uncus)
- Septal nuclei

This limbic ring links visceral states with conscious experience and behavioral responses.

Consolidated Narrative Summary Sheet

The cerebrum is the largest and most functionally sophisticated component of the human brain, housing most of the CNS neurons and serving as the seat of perception, voluntary movement, memory, language, emotion, and higher cognition. Although the hemispheres share a mirrored structural plan, certain functions, especially language and praxis—are lateralized.

External Organization

The hemispheres are separated by the interhemispheric fissure but interconnected by the corpus callosum, ensuring functional integration. The cerebral cortex forms a convoluted sheet of grey matter, while the underlying white matter contains association, commissural, and projection fibers. Deep nuclei such as the thalamus, basal nuclei, and amygdala contribute to sensory relay, motor modulation, and emotional processing.

Lobar Boundaries

- Central sulcus — separates frontal and parietal lobes
- Lateral sulcus — separates the temporal lobe from the frontal and parietal lobes
- Parieto-occipital sulcus — separates parietal and occipital lobes
- Preoccipital notch → parietooccipital sulcus line — defines anterior occipital boundary

Frontal Lobe

Contains the precentral gyrus (primary motor cortex), superior/middle/inferior frontal gyri, and Broca's area (pars opercularis + pars triangularis). The orbitofrontal surface includes the gyrus rectus and olfactory sulcus.

Parietal Lobe

Contains the postcentral gyrus (primary somatosensory cortex), postcentral sulcus, intraparietal sulcus, superior parietal lobule, and inferior parietal lobule (supramarginal and angular gyri).

Temporal Lobe

Is divided into superior, middle, and inferior temporal gyri. The inferior surface contains the occipitotemporal and collateral sulci, with the occipitotemporal gyrus between them. Medially lies the parahippocampal gyrus, uncus, and isthmus.

Occipital Lobe

Dominated by the calcarine sulcus and striate cortex. The cuneus lies above the calcarine sulcus; the lingual gyrus lies below it.

Limbic System

Includes the cingulate gyrus, subcallosal area, isthmus, parahippocampal gyrus, uncus, amygdala, and septal nuclei.

Review Questions

Q1. The central sulcus separates which two lobes?
Answer: Frontal and parietal lobes.

Q2. Which structure connects the right and left cerebral hemispheres?
Answer: Corpus callosum.

Q3. The primary visual cortex is located along which sulcus?
Answer: Calcarine sulcus.

Q4. The inferior frontal gyrus contains which language area in the dominant hemisphere?
Answer: Broca's area.

Q5. The parahippocampal gyrus curves medially to form which structure?
Answer: The uncus.

Q6. The supramarginal and angular gyri belong to which lobe?
Answer: Inferior parietal lobule of the parietal lobe.

Q7. The insula is hidden beneath which major sulcus?
Answer: Lateral sulcus.

Q8. The cuneus lies between which two sulci?
Answer: Parieto-occipital sulcus and calcarine sulcus.

Q9. The occipitotemporal gyrus lies between which two sulci?
Answer: Occipitotemporal sulcus and collateral sulcus.

References

1. Snell's Clinical Neuroanatomy
Snell RS. *Clinical Neuroanatomy*. 8th ed. Wolters Kluwer.

2. Gray's Anatomy for Students
Drake RL, Vogl W, Mitchell AWM. *Gray's Anatomy for Students*. 4th ed. Elsevier.

3. Neuroanatomy Through Clinical Cases
Blumenfeld H. *Neuroanatomy Through Clinical Cases*. 3rd ed. Sinauer Associates.

Chapter 6
Cerebrum: White matter

Click here to view
Chapter Video: https://youtu.be/Td__PhFdSlU

Overview

The cerebral white matter consists of an extensive network of myelinated nerve fibers that interconnect different regions of the brain. These fibers facilitate rapid communication between cortical areas, between the two cerebral hemispheres, and between the cerebral cortex and deeper structures such as the thalamus, brainstem, cerebellum, and spinal cord. Through these widespread pathways, white matter plays a central role in integrating sensory, motor, cognitive, and emotional functions.

Cerebral white matter fibers are organized into three principal systems. Association fibers connect cortical regions within the same hemisphere. Commissural fibers connect corresponding cortical areas of the two hemispheres. Projection fibers establish vertical connections between the cerebral cortex and subcortical and lower central nervous system structures. Together, these systems create an integrated network that supports normal neurological function.

Association Fibers

Association fibers interconnect cortical areas within the same cerebral hemisphere. They are classified into short and long association fibers.

Short association fibers, also called U fibers, lie immediately beneath the cerebral cortex and arch between adjacent gyri. These fibers provide rapid local communication and facilitate integration between neighboring cortical areas.

Long association fibers form major Intrahemispheric pathways that are essential for higher cortical functions such as language, memory, attention, emotional processing, and visuospatial integration. Damage to these pathways may produce characteristic neurological deficits. Lesions in the right hemisphere may lead to spatial hemineglect, whereas lesions in the dominant hemisphere may result in dysgraphia and other language-related impairments.

Major Long Association Bundles

The superior longitudinal fasciculus is a major association bundle that arches across the cerebral hemisphere and interconnects the frontal, parietal, temporal, and occipital lobes. A clinically important component of this fasciculus is the arcuate fasciculus, which connects Broca's area in the inferior frontal gyrus with Wernicke's area in the posterior temporal region. This pathway is essential for language repetition, verbal working memory, and integration of speech production with language comprehension. Damage to the arcuate fasciculus may result in conduction aphasia, a disorder characterized by fluent speech and preserved comprehension but impaired repetition.

The uncinate fasciculus is a hook-shaped bundle that extends from the orbitofrontal cortex to the anterior temporal lobe. It connects frontal cortical regions with limbic structures such as the amygdala and hippocampus and forms an important component of the ventral language pathway. It contributes to naming, semantic retrieval, emotional processing, and integration of memory with language. Injury to this tract may cause difficulty recognizing or naming familiar objects and faces.

Commissural Fibers

Commissural fibers cross the midline to connect corresponding cortical areas of the two cerebral hemispheres. They are essential for bilateral coordination of sensory, motor, and cognitive functions.

The corpus callosum is the largest commissural fiber bundle in the brain, containing approximately 200 to 800 million fibers. It forms the floor of the longitudinal cerebral fissure and serves as the principal pathway for interhemispheric communication. The rostrum primarily connects orbitofrontal regions, the genu interconnects prefrontal and premotor areas, the body connects motor and somatosensory cortices, and the splenium links occipital and visual association cortices. The splenium is particularly important for the transfer of visual information between the hemispheres and is essential for reading and visuospatial integration.

Other commissural pathways also contribute to interhemispheric communication. The anterior commissure lies near the lamina terminalis and interconnects olfactory regions, the amygdalae, and parts of the temporal lobes. The posterior commissure lies anterior to the pineal gland and is important in pupillary light reflex pathways. The fornix commissure, also known as the hippocampal commissure, interconnects the hippocampi and contributes to memory consolidation. The habenular commissure connects the habenular nuclei and participates in emotional and autonomic responses related to pain, stress, and reward.

Projection Fibers

Projection fibers establish vertical connections between the cerebral cortex and lower centers of the central nervous system. They connect the cortex with the thalamus, basal nuclei, brainstem, cerebellum, and spinal cord. These fibers include both ascending afferent pathways and descending efferent pathways.

Ascending projection fibers include thalamocortical pathways that relay sensory information, motor signals, and limbic input to the cerebral cortex. These fibers form an important part of the internal capsule and corona radiata and are essential for the transmission of information to higher cortical centers.

Descending projection fibers include several major motor pathways. The corticospinal tract is the principal voluntary motor pathway and controls movements of the trunk and limbs. The corticobulbar tract supplies the motor nuclei of cranial nerves and is responsible for functions such as facial expression, mastication, swallowing, and phonation.

Corticopontine fibers project from the cerebral cortex to the pontine nuclei, from where information is relayed to the cerebellum. These fibers form a major component of the cerebrocerebellar loop, which is essential for coordination of movement, motor planning, and motor learning.

Functional Significance

Association, commissural, and projection fibers together form an integrated communication network that enables the cerebral cortex to coordinate perception, movement, language, memory, emotion, and behavior. The structural and functional integrity of these white matter pathways is essential for normal neurological performance. Disruption of these pathways produces characteristic clinical syndromes that help localize lesions within the nervous system.

Review Questions

Q1. Damage to the arcuate fasciculus produces which clinical syndrome?
Answer: Conduction aphasia.

Q2. Which fiber system connects cortical areas within the same hemisphere?
Answer: Association fibers.

Q3. The splenium of the corpus callosum interconnects which cortical regions?
Answer: Visual cortices.

Q4. Injury to the right hemisphere's long association fibers may result in what deficit?
Answer: Spatial hemineglect.

Q5. Which commissure is involved in the pupillary light reflex?
Answer: Posterior commissure.

Q6. The uncinate fasciculus connects which major regions?
Answer: Orbitofrontal cortex with the amygdala and hippocampus.

Q7. Which projection fibers carry voluntary motor commands to the spinal cord?
Answer: Corticospinal tract.

Q8. The anterior commissure interconnects which structures?
Answer: Olfactory areas, amygdala, and temporal lobes.

Q9. Damage to area 43 results in loss of which sensation?
Answer: Taste (contralateral).

Q10. Thalamocortical fibers belong to which category of white matter pathways?
Answer: Projection fibers.

References

1. Kandel ER et al. *Principles of Neural Science.* 5th ed. McGraw-Hill; 2013.
2. Nolte J. *The Human Brain.* 7th ed. Elsevier; 2016.
3. Purves D et al. *Neuroscience.* 6th ed. Oxford University Press; 2018.
4. Standring S. *Gray's Anatomy.* 42nd ed. Elsevier; 2020.

Chapter 7

Cerebrum: Functional Areas

Click here to view
Chapter Video: https://youtu.be/5FIBOqTUfjM

Organization of Cortical Functional Areas

The cerebral cortex is the seat of all higher neurological functions. Every modality—motor, sensory, general, and special—is represented within its surface in a highly organized manner. Cortical functions are distributed across primary, secondary, and higher-order association areas, each contributing a distinct layer of processing.

- Primary areas receive raw sensory input or initiate motor output.
- Secondary areas refine, interpret, and contextualize this information.
- Association areas integrate multimodal inputs into meaningful perception, intention, and behavior.

This hierarchical arrangement underlies the cortex's ability to transform sensation into action and thought into purposeful movement.

Brodmann's Cytoarchitectonic Map

A foundational understanding of cortical functional anatomy begins with the work of Korbinian Brodmann, who used Nissl staining to identify regional variations in cortical layering. He divided the cortex into 52 Brodmann areas, a system that remains central to modern neuroanatomy and clinical localization.

These areas correlate strongly with functional domains such as motor control, somatosensory, vision, audition, and language.

Motor Cortex and Its Functional Subdivisions

The motor cortex occupies a substantial portion of the frontal lobe and includes:

- Primary motor cortex (Area 4) — precentral gyrus
- Premotor cortex (Area 6)
- Supplementary motor area (Area 6, medial surface)
- Frontal eye fields (Areas 8 and 9)
- Broca's speech region (Areas 44 and 45) in the dominant hemisphere

The primary motor cortex extends onto the medial surface as the anterior paracentral gyrus.

Somatotopic Organization: The Motor Homunculus

The body is represented on the primary motor cortex in a highly ordered somatotopic map known as the motor homunculus.

- Lower limb → medial surface
- Trunk and upper limb → superior and middle precentral gyrus
- Face and tongue → inferior margin

The head and neck are the only regions depicted upright.

The size of each cortical representation reflects precision and complexity, not anatomical size. Thus, the hand, face, and tongue occupy disproportionately large territories.

All motor output from the primary motor cortex influences the contralateral side of the body due to corticospinal decussation.

Hierarchy of Motor Planning and Execution

Motor function emerges from a coordinated sequence involving the secondary motor cortices:

Posterior Parietal Cortex (Areas 5 and 7)

- Integrates visual, proprioceptive, and spatial information
- Constructs the conceptual blueprint of intended movement

Supplementary Motor Area

- Selects and organizes motor programs
- Prepares the body for action
- Essential for bimanual coordination and internally generated movements

Premotor Cortex

- Translates the motor plan into a sequence of muscular activations
- Determines the order of agonist, antagonist, and synergist contractions
- Important for externally guided movements

Primary Motor Cortex

- Executes the final motor command via corticospinal neurons

This hierarchical flow—from conceptualization → planning → programming → execution—illustrates the sophistication of cortical motor control.

Clinical Correlates of Motor Cortex Lesions

Primary Motor Cortex Lesions

- Produce contralateral weakness or paralysis
- Deficits correspond to the somatotopic region affected
- Reflect loss of corticospinal output

Secondary Motor Cortex Lesions

- Do not cause paralysis
- Produce apraxia: inability to perform learned, purposeful movements despite intact strength and comprehension
- Highlight the role of premotor and supplementary areas in planning rather than force generation

Apraxia is a hallmark of frontal and parietal association cortex dysfunction.

Language Areas: Broca and Wernicke

Broca's Area (Areas 44 and 45)

Located in the inferior frontal gyrus of the dominant hemisphere, Broca's area is responsible for:

- Motor formulation of speech
- Word selection and phrase construction
- Coordination of articulatory movements

It communicates directly with the adjacent primary motor cortex controlling the larynx, tongue, lips, and palate.

Broca's aphasia (expressive aphasia):

- Slow, effortful, halting speech
- Comprehension relatively preserved
- Impaired fluency and sentence construction

Wernicke's Area

Located in the posterior superior temporal gyrus (dominant hemisphere), Wernicke's area mediates:

- Language comprehension
- Interpretation of spoken and written words

Wernicke's aphasia (receptive aphasia):

- Fluent but meaningless speech
- Impaired comprehension
- Paraphasias and neologisms

The contrast between expressive and receptive aphasia illustrates the division of labor between frontal and temporal language centers.

Frontal Eye Fields (Areas 8 and 9)

The frontal eye fields govern voluntary horizontal conjugate gaze.

- Enable the eyes to move together toward a chosen target
- Operate independently of visual stimuli

Lesion patterns:

- Irritative lesions (e.g., seizures) → eyes deviate away from the lesion
- Destructive lesions (e.g., stroke) → eyes deviate toward the lesion due to unopposed activity of the intact hemisphere

These deficits often improve as cortical control reorganizes.

Prefrontal, Parietal, Insular, Auditory, and Visual Cortices

Prefrontal Cortex: Executive and Emotional Regulation

Dorsolateral Prefrontal Cortex (Area 46)

The dorsolateral prefrontal cortex (DLPFC), located in the anterior frontal lobe, is the center of executive function. It supports:

- Working memory
- Planning and organization

- Judgment and abstract reasoning
- Inhibitory control
- Social behavior and decisionmaking

Damage from trauma, stroke, or degenerative disease may produce:
- Apathy and impaired initiative
- Personality changes
- Disinhibition
- Difficulty with complex problemsolving

Historically, prefrontal lobotomy targeted this region in misguided attempts to treat severe behavioral disorders—an approach now abandoned.

The DLPFC maintains reciprocal connections with the dorsomedial thalamic nucleus and amygdala, integrating cognition with emotion.

Orbitofrontal Cortex

The orbitofrontal cortex (OFC) contributes to:
- Emotional regulation
- Reward processing
- Social judgment
- Secondary taste perception

Lesions produce impulsive, socially inappropriate, or emotionally labile behavior, reflecting impaired inhibitory control.

Parietal Lobe: Somatosensory and Multimodal Integration

Primary Somatosensory Cortex (Areas 3, 1, 2)

Located between the central sulcus and postcentral sulcus, the primary somatosensory cortex receives thirdorder sensory neurons from the VPL and VPM nuclei of the thalamus.
- Area 3 (closest to central sulcus): principal receptive zone
- Area 1: texture and feature analysis
- Area 2: size, shape, and spatial discrimination

These areas form the cortical endpoint of the somatosensory pathways.
A lesion produces contralateral loss of tactile discrimination, vibration sense, and proprioception.

Cytoarchitecture

- Areas 3A and 3B → highly granular cortex with a prominent outer band of Baillarger
- Areas 1 and 2 → hypogranular, reflecting their integrative role

Secondary Somatosensory Areas (Areas 5 and 7)
Located in the superior parietal lobule, these areas integrate:

- Tactile input
- Proprioceptive signals
- Visual information

They construct a coherent representation of the body in space and guide movement.

Visuospatial Processing Regions

The region surrounding the intraparietal sulcus, along with the transitional zone between the parietal and occipital lobes, plays a central role in visuospatial processing.

Functions include:

- Identifying spatial relationships
- Integrating visual and proprioceptive input
- Locating objects relative to the body
- Guiding reaching and grasping

Damage produces:

- Impaired object recognition by shape or texture
- Difficulty localizing stimuli
- Inability to appreciate moving objects
- Disturbances in spatial awareness

Inferior Parietal Lobule: Language and Multimodal Integration
The inferior parietal lobule consists of:

- Supramarginal gyrus (Area 40)
- Angular gyrus (Area 39)

These gyri integrate auditory, visual, and somatosensory information.

In the dominant hemisphere, they are essential for:

- Language comprehension
- Reading (alexia when damaged)
- Writing (agraphia)
- Mathematical reasoning (acalculia)
- Body schema and spatial cognition

Lesions may produce Gerstmann syndrome (agraphia, acalculia, finger agnosia, leftright disorientation).

Primary Gustatory Cortex (Area 43)

Located in the upper bank of the posterior ramus of the lateral sulcus and the parietal operculum, Area 43 receives taste information from the thalamus.

Lesions cause contralateral loss of taste sensation.

Insular Cortex: Interoception and Emotional Integration

The insula, buried deep within the lateral sulcus, receives convergent input from sensory, limbic, autonomic, and prefrontal regions. It functions as a crossmodal integrative hub linking bodily states with emotional and cognitive experiences.

Anterior Insula

- Connected with the amygdala
- Processes emotional states: anger, fear, sadness, happiness
- Involved in sexual arousal and taste perception

Posterior Insula

- Receives input from the ventromedial thalamic nucleus
- Associated with the secondary somatosensory cortex
- Processes emotional aspects of:
  - Pain
  - Temperature
  - Itch
  - Sensual touch

Primary Auditory Cortex (Areas 41, 42, 22)

Located within the lateral sulcus and extending into the superior temporal gyrus, the primary auditory cortex performs the initial cortical processing of sound.

- Unilateral lesions → mild hearing impairment (due to bilateral projections)
- Bilateral lesions → cortical deafness

Primary Visual Cortex (Area 17, V1)

The primary visual cortex, or striate cortex, occupies the banks of the calcarine sulcus.

Key features:

- Six distinct layers
- Layer 4 receives most input from the lateral geniculate nucleus
- Stria of Gennari (outer band of Baillarger) gives V1 its striped appearance

Surrounding V1 are the Extrastriate visual areas:

- V2, V3 — form and contour
- V4 — color processing
- V5 (MT) — motion perception

Complete bilateral destruction of the occipital lobes produces cortical blindness.

Complete bilateral destruction of the primary visual cortex (Area 17) produces cortical blindness, a condition in which the eyes and optic pathways remain structurally intact, yet visual perception is absent due to loss of cortical processing. This deficit may be accompanied by anosognosia, a striking unawareness or denial of blindness known as Anton syndrome. Patients may insist they can see despite overwhelming evidence to the contrary, reflecting disruption of visual awareness networks in the occipital and parietal association cortices.

Review Questions

Q1. A lesion of Brodmann area 4 produces which deficit?
Answer: Contralateral weakness or paralysis due to loss of primary motor output.

Q2. Damage to the premotor cortex results in which condition?
Answer: Apraxia—an inability to perform learned movements despite intact strength.

Q3. A patient speaks slowly with effort but understands language well. Which area is affected?
Answer: Broca's area (expressive aphasia).

Q4. A patient produces fluent but meaningless speech and cannot understand spoken words. Which area is damaged?
Answer: Wernicke's area (receptive aphasia).

Q5. Irritative lesions of the frontal eye fields cause the eyes to deviate in which direction?
Answer: Toward the contralateral side.

Q6. Which Brodmann areas form the primary somatosensory cortex?
Answer: Areas 3, 1, and 2.

Q7. Lesions of the superior parietal lobule impair which function?
Answer: Visuospatial processing and integration of sensory modalities.

Q8. The supramarginal and angular gyri are essential for which cognitive functions?
Answer: Language comprehension, reading, writing, mathematical reasoning, and body schema.

Q9. Which cortical area serves as the primary gustatory cortex?
Answer: Area 43.

Q10. Bilateral lesions of the primary visual cortex produce what condition?
Answer: Cortical blindness.

Q11. What lesion causes conduction aphasia?
Answer: Arcuate fasciculus.

Q12. Which structure is essential for declarative memory consolidation?
Answer: Hippocampus.

Q13. A patient ignores the left side of space. Which lobe is affected?
Answer: Right parietal lobe.

Q14. Which cortical region regulates planning and inhibition?
Answer: Prefrontal cortex.

References

1. Kandel ER et al. *Principles of Neural Science.* 5th ed. McGraw-Hill; 2013.
2. Nolte J. *The Human Brain.* 7th ed. Elsevier; 2016.
3. Purves D et al. *Neuroscience.* 6th ed. Oxford University Press; 2018.
4. Standring S. *Gray's Anatomy.* 42nd ed. Elsevier; 2020.

Chapter 8

Gross Anatomy of the Brainstem 8 A -Midbrain, 8 B-Pons, 8 C -Medulla (Only video presentations - No text appended)

Click here to view

8 A - Midbrain video: https://youtu.be/O4zBZBTDOGw

8 B - Pons video: https://youtu.be/LyMwBrVy8Nc

8 C - Medulla video: https://youtu.be/x0zeEAZQaXI

Chapter 9

Reticular Formation & Consciousness

Click here to view
Chapter Video: https://youtu.be/DlmreZyulco

The reticular formation is a diffuse, netlike collection of neurons and fiber tracts that extends throughout the brainstem, from the medulla oblongata through the pons to the midbrain. It is strategically situated within the tegmentum and maintains extensive reciprocal connections with ascending and descending pathways, cranial nerve nuclei, the spinal cord, cerebellum, thalamus, hypothalamus, and cerebral cortex.

Unlike sharply defined nuclei, the reticular formation is composed of interconnected neuronal networks that form complex polysynaptic circuits. These circuits receive afferent input from nearly all sensory systems, with the notable exception of the dorsal column–medial lemniscal pathway, and project widely throughout the central nervous system. This extensive connectivity allows the reticular formation to function as a major integrative center for autonomic regulation, motor coordination, sensory modulation, pain control, and maintenance of consciousness.

Structural Organization of the Reticular Formation

The reticular formation is classically organized into three longitudinal functional zones.

The midline raphe nuclei are situated near the midline of the brainstem and represent the major source of serotonin within the central nervous system. Through their widespread projections, these nuclei play important roles in regulating mood, sleep, autonomic activity, and limbic function. They are also essential components of descending pain modulatory pathways.

The medial zone contains relatively large neurons with long ascending and descending axons. Functionally, this zone serves primarily as an output system. It gives rise to reticulospinal pathways that influence posture, muscle tone, and locomotion, and it integrates motor signals from the cerebral cortex and cerebellum.

The lateral zone contains smaller neurons and receives abundant afferent input. It functions primarily as an input-processing system, receiving sensory and visceral information, modulating cranial nerve reflexes, and regulating autonomic and visceral functions.

Medullary Reticular Formation

The medullary reticular formation contains several important nuclear groups that are essential for autonomic and reflex functions. These include the lateral nucleus, paramedian nucleus, ventral nucleus, magnocellular nucleus, and parvocellular nucleus.

Together, these nuclei form part of a central network responsible for respiratory rhythm generation, cardiovascular regulation, swallowing, vomiting, and postural reflexes. Their integrative role is crucial for maintaining internal homeostasis and coordinating vital brainstem functions.

Functional Roles of the Reticular Formation

Visceral and Autonomic Regulation

The reticular formation is a major regulator of autonomic homeostasis through its extensive connections with the hypothalamus, cranial parasympathetic nuclei, and sympathetic and parasympathetic spinal centers.

Through these pathways, the reticular formation regulates respiration by influencing medullary respiratory centers, phrenic motor neurons, and thoracic spinal cord neurons. It also modulates heart rate, regulates blood pressure and vasomotor tone, and coordinates visceral reflexes essential for internal physiological stability.

Motor Control and Postural Regulation

The reticular formation plays a major role in motor control via descending reticulospinal pathways. These pathways are essential for maintaining posture and equilibrium, regulating muscle tone, coordinating locomotion, and integrating vestibular, cerebellar, and corticospinal influences.

In addition, the reticular formation facilitates automatic and anticipatory postural adjustments that are necessary for smooth, coordinated movement and balance.

Pain Modulation

The reticular formation plays a critical role in descending pain control. Nociceptive signals from the spinal cord ascend through spinomesencephalic pathways to the periaqueductal gray matter and midbrain reticular formation.

The periaqueductal Gray then activates the raphe nuclei and medullary reticular formation. These structures send descending serotonergic and other modulatory fibers to the dorsal horn of the spinal cord, where interneurons suppress transmission of nociceptive signals.

This pathway forms an important component of the brain's intrinsic pain suppression system. The periaqueductal Gray contains a high density of opioid receptors, and both endogenous opioids, such as endorphins and enkephalins, and exogenous opioids exert their analgesic effects through this mechanism.

Ascending Reticular Activating System (ARAS)

The ascending reticular activating system is a functional network within the reticular formation that is essential for arousal, wakefulness, and maintenance of consciousness.

The ARAS receives multimodal sensory input from visual, auditory, vestibular, and somatosensory pathways. It also receives modulatory input from the hypothalamus, limbic system, and cerebral cortex.

From the brainstem, the ARAS projects diffusely to the intralaminar thalamic nuclei, hypothalamus, basal forebrain, and widespread regions of the cerebral cortex. These widespread projections maintain cortical activation, responsiveness, and vigilance.

Functionally, the ARAS is responsible for the maintenance of wakefulness, the regulation of sleep–wake transitions, the promotion of cortical alertness, the enhancement of attention, and the modulation of electroencephalographic activity from sleep to wakefulness.

Consciousness and the Reticular Formation

Consciousness depends on two major components: wakefulness, which refers to arousal, and awareness, which refers to the content of consciousness.

The reticular formation, particularly the ascending reticular activating system, provides the neurophysiological basis for wakefulness. Higher cortical and thalamic networks are responsible for generating awareness.

Wakefulness

Wakefulness is maintained through ARAS projections to the thalamus and cerebral cortex. Several brainstem neurotransmitter systems are involved in this process, including acetylcholine, norepinephrine, serotonin, dopamine, and histamine. These systems regulate cortical tone, attention, alertness, and behavioral responsiveness.

Awareness

Awareness depends on intact thalamocortical loops and functional cortical association networks. Integration across executive, salience, and default mode networks allows conscious perception, self-awareness, attention, and goal-directed behavior.

Clinical Correlation: Disorders of Consciousness

Disorders of consciousness reflect disruption of either wakefulness, awareness, or both. In a coma, both wakefulness and awareness are lost. This state usually results from severe bilateral cortical dysfunction or extensive injury to the ascending reticular activating system. In the vegetative state, wakefulness is preserved, as indicated by the presence of sleep–wake cycles, but awareness is absent. The minimally conscious state is characterized by intermittent but reproducible signs of awareness, with fluctuating responses to the environment.

Locked-in syndrome represents a unique clinical condition in which consciousness is preserved, but the patient is quadriplegic and unable to speak because of a ventral pontine lesion. Vertical eye movements may remain intact and provide a means of communication.

Lesions of the ascending reticular activating system have major clinical implications. Unilateral lesions usually produce relatively mild effects, whereas bilateral extensive lesions may result in stupor, coma, or irreversible loss of consciousness.

Functional Significance

The reticular formation is a central integrative system that coordinates autonomic regulation, sensory processing, motor control, pain modulation, and arousal. Its widespread connections allow it to influence nearly every level of the nervous system.

The medullary reticular formation supports vital reflexes such as respiration and cardiovascular control. Reticulospinal pathways maintain posture, muscle tone, and locomotion. Descending pathways from the periaqueductal Gray and raphe nuclei suppress pain transmission. The ascending reticular activating system sustains wakefulness and vigilance, while coordinated cortical and thalamic activity generates awareness.

A clear understanding of the reticular formation is essential for interpreting disorders of consciousness, autonomic dysfunction, postural abnormalities, and pain syndromes.

Review Questions

Q1. Which brainstem system maintains arousal and wakefulness?
Answer: Ascending Reticular Activating System (ARAS).

Q2. What neurotransmitter is primarily produced by raphe nuclei?
Answer: Serotonin.

Q3. Which tract from the RF helps maintain posture and balance?
Answer: Reticulospinal tract.

Q4. What is the clinical consequence of bilateral ARAS damage?
Answer: Irreversible coma.

Q5. How does the RF contribute to pain modulation?
Answer: Via descending inhibition from PAG → raphe nuclei → spinal cord.

Clinical Vignettes

Vignette 1 — ARAS Lesion
A patient with a brainstem stroke is unresponsive, with no sleep–wake cycles.
Diagnosis: Coma due to ARAS damage.

Vignette 2 — Vegetative State
A patient opens eyes and shows sleep–wake cycles but no purposeful behavior.
Diagnosis: Vegetative state.

Vignette 3 — Pain Modulation
A patient receives morphine for severe pain.
Explanation: Exogenous opiates act on PAG receptors, mimicking endogenous pain suppression.

Vignette 4 — Reticulospinal Dysfunction: A patient with pontine hemorrhage shows severe postural instability.
Localization: Reticulospinal tract involvement.

References

1. Snell's Clinical Neuroanatomy
Snell RS. *Clinical Neuroanatomy*. 8th ed. Wolters Kluwer.

2. Gray's Anatomy for Students
Drake RL, Vogl W, Mitchell AWM. *Gray's Anatomy for Students*. 4th ed. Elsevier.

3. Neuroanatomy Through Clinical Cases
Blumenfeld H. *Neuroanatomy Through Clinical Cases*. 3rd ed. Sinauer Associates.

Chapter 10
Spinal Cord

Click here to view
Chapter Video: https://youtu.be/LFnMO9qxcC8

Introduction

The spinal cord is the caudal continuation of the central nervous system and begins at the inferior border of the medulla oblongata, just below the foramen magnum. Although it is continuous with the brainstem, it possesses a distinct internal organization and functional architecture. The emergence of the first cervical spinal nerve marks the anatomical transition between the brainstem and spinal cord.

Cylindrical in shape, the spinal cord measures approximately 45 cm in length and 1 to 1.5 cm in diameter. It occupies the upper two-thirds of the vertebral canal and terminates as the conus medullaris, usually at the level of the first lumbar vertebra in adults. This termination level reflects the differential growth rates of the spinal cord and vertebral column during development.

Segmental Organization

The spinal cord is divided into thirty-one segments, each of which gives rise to a pair of spinal nerves. These include eight cervical, twelve thoracic, five lumbar, five sacral, and one coccygeal segment. Although the spinal cord itself ends at the L1 vertebral level in adults, the lumbar, sacral, and coccygeal nerve roots continue inferiorly within the dural sac before exiting through their respective intervertebral foramina. This elongated bundle of nerve roots forms the cauda equina, a clinically important structure in lumbar puncture and cauda equina syndrome.

Surface Features of the Spinal Cord

The spinal cord displays several longitudinal grooves and sulci that serve as important anatomical landmarks.

On the dorsal surface, the posterior median sulcus forms a shallow midline depression. A fibrous septum extends inward from this sulcus and partially divides the dorsal white matter. The dorsolateral sulcus marks the entry point of dorsal sensory rootlets.

On the ventral surface, the anterior median fissure forms a prominent groove along the midline. This fissure is separated from the central Gray matter by the anterior white commissure, which contains decussating fibers. The ventrolateral sulcus marks the exit of ventral motor rootlets.

These surface features are essential for understanding the organization of spinal pathways and root entry zones.

Cervical and Lumbosacral Enlargements

The spinal cord exhibits two symmetrical enlargements that reflect increased neuronal density required for limb innervation.

The cervical enlargement extends from C5 to T1 and contributes to the brachial plexus, which supplies the upper limb. The lumbosacral enlargement extends from L1 to S3 and gives rise to the lumbosacral plexus, which innervates the lower limb.

Exit of Spinal Nerves

The pattern of spinal nerve exit has important clinical relevance. The first cervical spinal nerve exits above the C1 vertebra, and this pattern continues through C7. The C8 spinal nerve exits below the C7 vertebra, despite the absence of a corresponding C8 vertebra. From T1 downward, all spinal nerves exit below their corresponding vertebrae.

Certain sacral and coccygeal nerves show exceptions to this pattern. The S5 and coccygeal nerves exit through the sacral hiatus, while the anterior and posterior divisions of the sacral nerves pass through the sacral foramina.

Developmental Descent of the Spinal Cord

During early fetal development, the spinal cord extends the full length of the vertebral canal. As development progresses, the vertebral column grows more rapidly than the spinal cord, causing the spinal cord to appear to ascend.

At birth, the spinal cord usually ends at the level of L3, whereas in adults it ends at L1. This developmental change explains the formation of the cauda equina and the relative safety of performing a lumbar puncture below the L3 level.

Meningeal Coverings of the Spinal Cord

The spinal cord is enclosed by three protective meningeal layers: the dura mater, arachnoid mater, and pia mater. Together, these layers provide mechanical protection and maintain the cerebrospinal fluid environment.

The dura mater is the tough, fibrous outer covering. It extends from the foramen magnum to the level of S2, forming the dural sac. The dura mater is separated from the vertebral canal by the epidural space, which contains the internal vertebral venous plexus, adipose tissue, and loose areolar tissue.

The arachnoid mater is a thin, avascular membrane that lies deep to the dura. It is separated from the pia mater by the subarachnoid space, which contains cerebrospinal fluid and arachnoid trabeculae. The arachnoid terminates at S2. Inferior to the conus medullaris, the subarachnoid space expands to form the lumbar cistern, which contains the cauda equina and a substantial portion of total cerebrospinal fluid.

The pia mater is the innermost meningeal layer and closely adheres to the surface of the spinal cord. It extends along the nerve roots and forms specialized supporting structures.

The filum terminale is a slender extension of the pia mater that provides longitudinal stability. Its internal part extends from the conus medullaris to S2, while the external part pierces the dura and anchors to the coccyx.

Denticulate ligaments are lateral tooth-like extensions of the pia mater that anchor the spinal cord to the dura and help maintain its central position within the subarachnoid space.

Lumbar Puncture and Epidural Anesthesia

Lumbar puncture is performed for diagnostic and therapeutic purposes, including cerebrospinal fluid pressure measurement, biochemical and cytological analysis, spinal anesthesia, intrathecal drug administration, and myelography.

The procedure is usually performed in the lumbar region, where the needle passes sequentially through the skin, superficial fascia, supraspinous ligament, interspinous ligament, ligamentum flavum, epidural space, dura mater, and arachnoid mater before entering the cerebrospinal fluid within the subarachnoid space.

Epidural anesthesia involves the injection of an anesthetic into the epidural space, often through the sacral hiatus. This technique targets lower lumbar and sacral nerve roots and is widely used for painless childbirth and pelvic procedures.

Internal Architecture of the Spinal Cord

A transverse section of the spinal cord reveals centrally located Gray matter surrounded by white matter.

Gray Matter

The Gray matter forms an H-shaped central core and contains neuronal cell bodies, dendrites, synapses, and supporting neuroglia. It is divided into dorsal horns, ventral horns, and lateral horns.

The dorsal horns are primarily involved in sensory processing. The ventral horns contain somatic motor neurons that innervate skeletal muscle. The lateral horns contain autonomic neurons, with sympathetic preganglionic neurons located from T1 to L2 and parasympathetic preganglionic neurons from S2 to S4.

The central canal lies at the center of the Gray matter and is continuous superiorly with the fourth ventricle.

Rexed Laminae

The spinal Gray matter is functionally subdivided into ten Rexed laminae.

Laminae I to VI occupy the dorsal horn and are primarily concerned with sensory processing. Lamina I, also called the Dorsomarginal nucleus, receives pain and temperature fibers. Lamina II, the substantia gelatinosa, is a major site of nociceptive modulation. Laminae III and IV form the nucleus proprius and process pain, temperature, pressure, and vibration, while contributing to spinothalamic pathways. Laminae V and VI, especially prominent in cervical and lumbosacral enlargements, receive afferents from deep tissues, joints, and muscles.

Lamina VII forms the intermediate zone and plays a major role in autonomic regulation and proprioceptive integration. It contains the nucleus dorsalis of Clarke from C8 to L4, which receives proprioceptive input and gives rise to the ipsilateral dorsal spinocerebellar tract. It also contains the intermediolateral cell column, which houses sympathetic and parasympathetic preganglionic neurons.

Lamina VIII contains interneurons involved in reflex integration and receives vestibulospinal and reticulospinal input. Lamina IX contains alpha and gamma motor neurons arranged in medial and lateral motor groups. Lamina X surrounds the central canal and contains decussating interneurons involved in bilateral reflexes, visceral pain transmission, and pelvic organ reflexes.

White Matter

The white matter surrounds the Gray matter and contains ascending and descending fiber tracts organized into posterior, lateral, and anterior columns.

The posterior columns contain the fasciculus gracilis and fasciculus cuneatus, which transmit fine touch, vibration, and conscious proprioception. The lateral columns contain major ascending and descending tracts, including the spinothalamic tract, corticospinal tract, and spinocerebellar pathways. The anterior columns contain motor pathways and reticulospinal fibers.

The anterior white commissure contains decussating fibers, including those of the spinothalamic pathway.

Vascular Supply of the Spinal Cord

The spinal cord receives its blood supply from three longitudinal arteries reinforced by segmental feeder vessels.

The anterior spinal artery is formed by branches of the vertebral arteries and descends in the anterior median fissure. It supplies the anterior two-thirds of the spinal cord, including the corticospinal tracts, spinothalamic tracts, and ventral horns.

Two posterior spinal arteries descend along the dorsolateral sulci and supply the posterior one-third of the spinal cord, including the fasciculus gracilis and fasciculus cuneatus.

Segmental reinforcement is provided by anterior segmental medullary arteries, ascending cervical arteries, intercostal arteries, the artery of Adamkiewicz, and branches of the iliolumbar artery. Typically, a major feeder vessel reinforces the cord every four to six segments.

Clinical Correlates: Spinal Cord Vascular Syndromes

Occlusion of the anterior spinal artery or its feeder arteries produces anterior spinal artery syndrome, resulting in ischemia of the anterior two-thirds of the spinal cord. Clinically, this presents with bilateral upper motor neuron weakness below the lesion, loss of pain and temperature sensation due to spinothalamic tract involvement, and autonomic dysfunction. Dorsal column functions such as proprioception, vibration sense, and fine touch are usually preserved.

Occlusion of the posterior spinal arteries primarily affects the dorsal columns and results in ipsilateral loss of proprioception, vibration sense, and tactile discrimination. Motor pathways and spinothalamic tracts are generally spared.

Review Questions

Q1. A lumbar puncture at L4–L5 avoids which structure?
Answer: Spinal cord (ends at L1).

Q2. A lesion of the intermediolateral cell column (T1–L2) impairs what?
Answer: Sympathetic outflow.

Q3. Loss of vibration and proprioception on the right below T10 suggests occlusion of which artery?
Answer: Right posterior spinal artery.

Q4. Which nucleus gives rise to the dorsal spinocerebellar tract?
Answer: Clarke's nucleus (lamina VII).

Q5. The dorsal root enters the spinal cord at which landmark?
Answer: Dorsolateral sulcus.

Q6. Lamina II is responsible for which modality?
Answer: Pain modulation (substantia gelatinosa).

Q7. Lateral motor neurons of lamina IX innervate what?
Answer: Limb musculature.

Q8. Bilateral loss of pain and temperature with preserved proprioception indicates which syndrome?
Answer: Anterior spinal artery syndrome.

Q9. The filum terminale externum attaches to what?
Answer: Coccyx.

Q10. Which structure stabilizes the spinal cord laterally?
Answer: Denticulate ligaments.

Q11. The artery of Adamkiewicz reinforces which region?
Answer: Lower thoracic and upper lumbar cord.

Q12. Which lamina receives afferents from deep muscles and joints?
Answer: Laminae V and VI.

Q13. A ventral horn lesion produces what deficit?
Answer: Lower motor neuron weakness at the level of the lesion.

Q14. The anterior white commissure contains fibers of which pathway?
Answer: Spinothalamic tract.

Q15. The cauda equina is located in which space?
Answer: Lumbar cistern (subarachnoid space).

References

1. Standring S. *Gray's Anatomy.* 42nd ed. Elsevier; 2020.
2. Nolte J. *The Human Brain.* 7th ed. Elsevier; 2016.
3. Blumenfeld H. *Neuroanatomy Through Clinical Cases.* 3rd ed. Sinauer Associates; 2021.
4. Waxman SG. *Clinical Neuroanatomy.* 29th ed. McGraw-Hill; 2020.

Chapter 11

Ventricles of the Brain and Cerebrospinal Fluid: Anatomy, Development, Circulation, and Functional Significance

---

Click here to view
Chapter Video: https://youtu.be/IKaN7s1tw5M

Introduction

The ventricular system is a series of interconnected, ependymal-lined cavities derived from the embryonic neural tube. These chambers contain cerebrospinal fluid (CSF), a clear and colorless fluid that is essential for mechanical protection, metabolic stability, and homeostatic regulation of the central nervous system. The ventricular system consists of the two lateral ventricles, the third ventricle, and the fourth ventricle, which communicate through narrow channels that permit continuous circulation of CSF from its sites of production to its sites of reabsorption.

Development and General Organization

During embryonic development, the neural tube undergoes differential expansion, giving rise to the ventricular system. The telencephalon forms the lateral ventricles, the diencephalon forms the third ventricle, the mesencephalon gives rise to the cerebral aqueduct, and the rhombencephalon develops into the fourth ventricle. This embryological origin explains the close anatomical relationship between the ventricular cavities and the surrounding brain structures.

Each ventricle contains a choroid plexus, a specialized vascular and ependymal structure responsible for producing most of the CSF. Although the total CSF volume present within the central nervous system at any given time is approximately 150 mL, the choroid plexus produces nearly 500 to 600 mL each day, reflecting the dynamic turnover of this fluid.

Anatomy of the Ventricular System

Lateral Ventricles

The lateral ventricles are paired C-shaped cavities situated within the cerebral hemispheres. Each ventricle is divided into an anterior horn extending into the frontal lobe, a body located in the frontal and parietal lobes, a posterior horn extending into the occipital lobe, an inferior horn projecting into the temporal lobe, and a trigone or atrium located at the junction of the body with the three horns. These ventricles communicate with the third ventricle through the interventricular foramina, also known as the foramina of Monro.

Third Ventricle

The third ventricle is a narrow midline cavity located within the diencephalon. Its lateral walls are formed mainly by the thalami, while the inferolateral boundaries are related to the hypothalamus. The ventricle is lined by ependymal cells and contains a choroid plexus within its roof. In many individuals, the cavity is partially bridged by the interthalamic adhesion. Anteriorly, it communicates with the lateral ventricles through the foramina of Monro, and posteriorly, it continues into the cerebral aqueduct.

Fourth Ventricle

The fourth ventricle lies dorsal to the pons and upper medulla and ventral to the cerebellum. It has a tent-shaped cavity lined by ependymal cells and contains paired choroid plexuses. Superiorly, it communicates with the cerebral aqueduct, and inferiorly, it continues with the central canal of the spinal cord.

Cerebrospinal fluid exits the fourth ventricle into the subarachnoid space through one median aperture, the foramen of Magendie, and two lateral apertures, the foramina of Luschka. Obstruction of these outlets, particularly by posterior fossa tumors or congenital malformations, can produce non-communicating hydrocephalus.

Cerebrospinal Fluid: Production and Circulation

Production of CSF

Cerebrospinal fluid is produced primarily by the choroid plexus, which consists of fenestrated capillaries covered by specialized choroid epithelial cells derived from ependyma. CSF formation occurs mainly through active transport of sodium ions, followed by chloride and water movement across the epithelium. In addition to water and electrolytes, the choroid plexus transports hormones, peptides, growth factors, micronutrients, and complement proteins into the CSF.

CSF secretion occurs at an approximate rate of 20 to 25 mL per hour, producing a total daily volume of 500 to 600 mL, while the total circulating volume remains about 150 mL. The ependymal lining of the ventricles and central canal also produces a smaller amount of CSF.

Circulation of CSF

Cerebrospinal fluid follows a well-defined pathway. It is produced within the lateral ventricles, passes through the foramina of Monro into the third ventricle, and then flows through the cerebral aqueduct into the fourth ventricle. From there, it exits through the foramina of Luschka and Magendie into the subarachnoid space surrounding the brain and spinal cord. Ultimately, it is reabsorbed into the venous circulation through arachnoid granulations, especially into the superior sagittal sinus.

Reabsorption of CSF

CSF is reabsorbed mainly through arachnoid villi and granulations that project into the dural venous sinuses. This process is pressure-dependent and helps maintain a stable intracranial pressure and constant CSF volume.

Functions of Cerebrospinal Fluid

Cerebrospinal fluid performs several essential physiological functions.

Its mechanical protective role allows it to cushion the brain and spinal cord against trauma. By suspending the brain within the cranial cavity, CSF reduces the effective weight of the brain by approximately 95 percent, thereby minimizing pressure on the basal structures.

CSF also maintains chemical stability within the extracellular environment of the central nervous system. It helps regulate ionic balance, provides nutrients, and facilitates the removal of metabolic waste products.

In addition, CSF serves as a transport medium for hormones, neurotransmitters, releasing factors, and signaling molecules, thereby contributing to communication between the central nervous system and systemic circulation.

CSF further acts as an environmental interface that supports immune surveillance, homeostasis, and maintenance of the specialized internal milieu required for neuronal function.

CSF Composition and Comparison with Plasma

Although cerebrospinal fluid is often compared with plasma, it is not a simple ultrafiltrate. Rather, it is a selectively produced fluid with a distinct biochemical composition regulated by active transport and barrier mechanisms.

Compared with plasma, CSF contains significantly lower protein levels, lower concentrations of potassium and calcium, and relatively higher chloride concentration. Its composition reflects the specialized ionic environment required for synaptic transmission and neuronal excitability.

The blood–CSF barrier, while less restrictive than the blood–brain barrier, remains highly selective and plays a critical role in preserving CNS homeostasis.

Lumbar Puncture and Clinical Relevance

Lumbar puncture is a diagnostic and therapeutic procedure performed to obtain cerebrospinal fluid from the lumbar cistern.

The preferred site of needle insertion is the L3–L4 or L4–L5 intervertebral space. This location is chosen because it lies below the termination of the spinal cord, thereby minimizing the risk of direct neural injury.

Lumbar puncture is commonly indicated in suspected meningitis, suspected subarachnoid hemorrhage, evaluation of demyelinating disorders, measurement of CSF opening pressure, and therapeutic drainage in selected cases such as idiopathic intracranial hypertension.

Important contraindications include raised intracranial pressure due to the risk of brain herniation, local infection at the puncture site, and bleeding disorders or anticoagulation therapy.

Clinical Significance

A sound understanding of the ventricular system and CSF physiology is essential for recognizing neurological disorders such as hydrocephalus, meningitis, intracranial hemorrhage, and disorders of CSF circulation. The ventricular system is not merely a passive set of cavities; it is a dynamic and highly regulated system that protects, nourishes, and supports the central nervous system.

Review Questions

Q1. Which structure connects the lateral ventricles to the third ventricle?
Answer: Interventricular foramina of Monro.

Q2. Through which openings do CSF exit the fourth ventricle?
Answer: Foramen of Magendie and foramina of Luschka.

Q3. What is the total volume of CSF in the CNS at any given time?
Answer: Approximately 150 ml.

Q4. What is the primary site of CSF reabsorption?
Answer: Arachnoid granulations in the superior sagittal sinus.

Clinical Vignette

A 7-year-old child presents with headache, vomiting, and gait instability. MRI reveals a midline posterior fossa tumor compressing the roof of the fourth ventricle. The foramina of Magendie and Luschka are obstructed.

Diagnosis: Noncommunicating (obstructive) hydrocephalus
Explanation: Obstruction of the fourth ventricular apertures prevents CSF from entering the subarachnoid space, causing dilation of the ventricles proximal to the blockage. This leads to increased intracranial pressure and the classic triad of headache, vomiting, and gait disturbance.

References

1. Snell's Clinical Neuroanatomy
Snell RS. *Clinical Neuroanatomy*. 8th ed. Wolters Kluwer.

2. Gray's Anatomy for Students
Drake RL, Vogl W, Mitchell AWM. *Gray's Anatomy for Students*. 4th ed. Elsevier.

3. Neuroanatomy Through Clinical Cases
Blumenfeld H. *Neuroanatomy Through Clinical Cases*. 3rd ed. Sinauer Associates.

Chapter 12

Thalamus: Gross Anatomy, Functional Overview, and Nuclear Organization

Click here to view
Chapter Video: https://youtu.be/q02UziQaluE

Introduction and Functional Significance

The thalamus is the largest component of the diencephalon and occupies a central position within the sensory and motor networks of the brain. It serves as the principal relay station for nearly all sensory information ascending to the cerebral cortex, with olfaction being the major exception. In addition to its sensory relay role, the thalamus participates in motor planning and execution through its connections with the basal ganglia and cerebellum, regulates arousal and consciousness through its links with the reticular activating system, modulates nociceptive pathways, and contributes to memory, emotion, executive function, and cognition. Because of its extensive reciprocal connections with the cerebral cortex, limbic system, basal ganglia, and brainstem, lesions of the thalamus can produce widespread neurological deficits.

Each thalamus is an ovoid mass of grey matter located on either side of the third ventricle. It tapers anteriorly and expands posteriorly into the pulvinar, a prominent posterior projection. Superiorly, the thalamus forms part of the floor of the lateral ventricle and is related to the choroid plexus and fornix. Inferiorly, it is separated from the hypothalamus by the hypothalamic sulcus. Medially, it forms the lateral wall of the third ventricle. Laterally, it is related superiorly to the caudate nucleus and inferiorly to the internal capsule. Posteriorly, it is continuous with the subthalamic region, which separates it from the midbrain. These anatomical relationships are of major clinical importance in understanding vascular syndromes, mass lesions, and neurosurgical approaches.

Functionally, the thalamus is indispensable for the relay of somatosensory, visual, auditory, gustatory, and visceral signals to the cortex. It also acts as an integrative center for motor activity through its interactions with the basal ganglia and cerebellar systems. In addition, it modulates pain perception, supports wakefulness and consciousness, and plays a key role in emotional behavior and memory through its limbic connections. Its central position within cortical and subcortical networks makes it essential for coordinated brain function.

The internal organization of the thalamus is defined by the internal medullary lamina, a Y-shaped sheet of white matter that divides the thalamus into anterior, medial, and lateral nuclear groups. The external surfaces of the thalamus are also covered by thin layers of white matter. This structural arrangement forms the basis for the functional specialization of thalamic nuclei.

The anterior nuclear group is enclosed within the anterior bifurcation of the internal medullary lamina. This group is an important component of the limbic system. It receives afferent input from the hippocampal formation through the fornix and from the mammillary bodies via the mammillothalamic tract. Its efferent fibers project mainly to the cingulate gyrus. Through these connections, the anterior nucleus forms an essential part of the Papez circuit and is involved in memory consolidation, emotional processing, and learning. Lesions affecting this nucleus may lead to anterograde amnesia and disturbances in emotional regulation.

The medial nuclear group is dominated by the dorsomedial, or mediodorsal, nucleus. This nucleus has extensive reciprocal connections with the prefrontal cortex and limbic structures. It is involved in emotional regulation, memory, motivation, judgment, personality, and the integration of somatic and visceral responses. Because of its role in higher cortical function, lesions of the mediodorsal nucleus may produce apathy, emotional blunting, impaired decision-making, disinhibition, and personality changes.

The lateral nuclear group is the largest division of the thalamus and is subdivided into dorsal and ventral tiers. The dorsal tier includes the lateral dorsal nucleus, lateral posterior nucleus, pulvinar, and the geniculate bodies. The lateral dorsal nucleus has limbic associations and contributes to emotional integration. The lateral posterior nucleus maintains reciprocal connections with the posterior parietal cortex and participates in spatial awareness, higher-order visual processing, and multimodal sensory integration. Together with the pulvinar, it forms part of the parietotemporal-occipital association network, which transforms sensory inputs into coherent perceptual experiences.

The pulvinar is the largest thalamic nucleus and forms the expanded posterior part of the thalamus. It has extensive reciprocal connections with the parietal, temporal, and occipital association cortices. Through these pathways, it integrates visual, auditory, and somatosensory information and supports attention, language-related functions, and higher-order perceptual processing. Lesions of the pulvinar may result in spatial hemineglect, attentional deficits, and impaired visual integration.

The ventral tier of the lateral nuclear group contains the principal motor and somatosensory relay nuclei. These are arranged from anterior to posterior as the ventral anterior (VA), ventral lateral (VL), and ventral posterior (VP) nuclei. The ventral posterior nucleus is further subdivided into the ventral posterior lateral (VPL), ventral posterior medial (VPM), and ventral posterior inferior (VPI) nuclei.

The ventral anterior nucleus is a major motor relay nucleus. It receives afferent fibers primarily from the globus pallidus and substantia nigra and projects to the premotor cortex and supplementary motor area. It is involved in motor planning and initiation of voluntary movement.

The ventral lateral nucleus is another important motor relay nucleus. It receives cerebellar afferents, especially from the dentate nucleus, and projects to the primary motor cortex, supplementary motor area, and premotor cortex. Through the dentatothalamocortical pathway, the VL nucleus conveys cerebellar feedback required for coordination, precision, and timing of movement.

The ventral posterior lateral nucleus receives somatosensory input from the contralateral body through the medial lemniscus and spinothalamic tracts. It relays this information to the primary somatosensory cortex in Brodmann areas 3, 1, and 2. The ventral posterior medial nucleus receives trigeminal lemniscal fibers carrying sensation from the face and gustatory fibers carrying taste information. It also projects to the primary somatosensory cortex and gustatory cortical areas. The ventral posterior inferior nucleus receives vestibulothalamic fibers and projects to vestibular cortical regions, contributing to balance, posture, and spatial orientation.

The lateral geniculate nucleus is the primary visual relay nucleus of the thalamus. It receives retinal input through the optic tract and projects to the primary visual cortex in Brodmann area 17. The medial geniculate nucleus is the primary auditory relay nucleus. It receives afferent fibers from the inferior colliculus and projects to the primary auditory cortex in Brodmann areas 41 and 42. These nuclei are essential for the cortical perception of visual and auditory stimuli.

The intralaminar nuclei are located within the internal medullary lamina and receive input from the reticular formation, trigeminal pain pathways, and basal ganglia. They are involved in arousal, alertness, pain modulation, and the ascending reticular activating system. These nuclei help maintain wakefulness and contribute to diffuse cortical activation.

Surrounding the lateral aspect of the thalamus is the thalamic reticular nucleus, a thin shell of GABAergic inhibitory neurons. This nucleus receives collateral input from both thalamocortical and corticothalamic fibers and provides inhibitory feedback to other thalamic nuclei. It plays a critical role in sensory gating, selective attention, and regulation of sleep rhythms, particularly sleep spindles. Dysfunction of the reticular nucleus has been implicated in epilepsy, schizophrenia, and attention disorders.

The thalamus also contains important association nuclei, particularly the mediodorsal nucleus and the pulvinar–lateral posterior complex. These nuclei contribute to executive function, motivation, emotional regulation, decision-making, and multimodal integration. Through their reciprocal cortical connections, they enable higher cognitive functions and perceptual coherence.

Lesions of specific thalamic nuclei produce characteristic clinical syndromes. Damage to the VPL or VPM nuclei results in contralateral loss of pain, temperature, touch, and proprioception. In some cases, this may progress to central post-stroke pain syndrome, also known as thalamic pain syndrome. Lesions of the lateral geniculate nucleus may cause contralateral homonymous hemianopia. Damage to the medial geniculate nucleus may result in diminished hearing and impaired sound localization. Lesions of the mediodorsal nucleus may produce apathy, emotional blunting, and personality changes. Injury to the anterior nucleus can impair memory. Pulvinar lesions may cause neglect syndromes and attentional deficits. Disruption of thalamocortical language pathways may lead to thalamic aphasia.

The vascular supply of the thalamus is derived from branches of the posterior circulation. The polar, or tuberothalamic, artery usually arises from the posterior communicating artery and supplies the anterior thalamus. The Thalamoperforating arteries arise from the P1 segment of the posterior cerebral artery and supply the paramedian region. The thalamogeniculate arteries arise from the P2 segment and supply the lateral thalamus. The posterior choroidal arteries also arise from the P2 segment and supply the posterior thalamus and pulvinar.

Occlusion of these vessels produces characteristic stroke syndromes. Polar artery infarction may present with apathy, aphasia, and acute amnesia. Thalamoperforating artery infarction may cause altered consciousness, behavioral changes, and vertical gaze palsy. Thalamogeniculate artery infarction often produces contralateral sensory loss, ataxia, and central pain syndrome. Posterior choroidal artery infarction may result in visual field deficits, impaired smooth pursuit eye movements, visual hallucinations, and psychiatric symptoms.

In summary, the thalamus is the central integrative hub of the forebrain, linking sensory input, motor control, consciousness, emotion, and cognition. Its highly organized nuclear architecture and extensive cortical and subcortical connections make it indispensable for normal neurological function. A clear understanding of thalamic anatomy and function is therefore essential for interpreting both normal brain physiology and the clinical manifestations of thalamic disease.

Review Questions

Q1. Which thalamic nucleus relays somatosensory information from the body?
Answer: Ventral posterior lateral (VPL).

Q2. A lesion of the medial geniculate nucleus produces what deficit?
Answer: Impaired hearing and difficulty localizing sound.

Q3. Which nucleus receives cerebellar dentate input?
Answer: Ventral lateral (VL) nucleus.

Q4. The anterior nucleus participates in which major limbic circuit?
Answer: Papez circuit.

Q5. Which thalamic nucleus is most associated with personality and executive function?
Answer: Dorsomedial (mediodorsal) nucleus.

Q6. A lesion of the pulvinar produces what deficit?
Answer: Spatial hemineglect and attentional impairment.

Q7. Which artery supplies the anterior thalamus?
Answer: Polar (tuberothalamic) artery.

Q8. What is the primary function of the reticular nucleus of the thalamus?
Answer: Inhibitory modulation of thalamocortical activity.

Clinical Vignettes

Vignette 1 — Sensory Loss
A 62-year-old man presents with numbness and loss of vibration sense on the right side of his body. Pain and temperature are also diminished. MRI shows a left thalamic infarct.
Affected nucleus: Ventral posterior lateral (VPL).

Vignette 2 — Behavioral Change
A 55-year-old woman becomes apathetic, emotionally indifferent, and poorly motivated after a stroke. No motor or sensory deficits.
Affected nucleus: Dorsomedial (mediodorsal) nucleus.

Vignette 3 — Visual Deficit
A patient with a PCA stroke presents with contralateral homonymous hemianopia.
Affected structure: Lateral geniculate nucleus (LGN).

Vignette 4 — Motor Dysfunction
A 48-year-old man has difficulty initiating voluntary movements despite normal strength. Imaging shows a lesion receiving pallidal input.
Affected nucleus: Ventral anterior (VA) nucleus.

Vignette 5 — Thalamic Pain Syndrome
A patient develops severe burning pain on one side of the body weeks after a thalamic stroke.
Likely artery occluded: Thalamogeniculate artery.

Vignette 6 — Spatial Neglect
A patient ignores objects in the left visual field and fails to respond to stimuli on that side.
Affected nucleus: Pulvinar.

Vignette 7 — Altered Consciousness
A 70-year-old patient presents with sudden confusion, somnolence, and vertical gaze palsy. Imaging shows a paramedian thalamic infarct.
Likely vessel: Thalamic/subthalamic (paramedian) artery.

References

1. Gray's Anatomy for Students
   Drake RL, Vogl W, Mitchell AWM. *Gray's Anatomy for Students*. 4th ed. Elsevier.
2. Neuroanatomy Through Clinical Cases
   Blumenfeld H. *Neuroanatomy Through Clinical Cases*. 3rd ed. Sinauer Associates.
3. Principles of Neural Science
   Kandel ER, et al. *Principles of Neural Science*. 6th ed. McGraw-Hill.

Chapter 13

Hypothalamus: Gross Anatomy, Functional Overview, and Zonal Organization

Click here to view
Chapter Video: https://youtu.be/DXkts1eO4_k

Introduction and Functional Significance

The hypothalamus is a major derivative of the diencephalon and lies immediately inferior to the thalamus, forming a substantial part of the walls and floor of the third ventricle. Although small in size, it exerts profound influence over nearly every aspect of internal physiology and is regarded as the principal neuroendocrine and autonomic integration center of the body. Through extensive neural and hormonal connections, the hypothalamus maintains homeostasis by regulating thermoregulation, hunger and satiety, circadian rhythms, reproductive behavior, emotional responses, blood pressure, electrolyte balance, and energy metabolism. Its intimate control over the pituitary gland enables it to coordinate both rapid autonomic responses and long-term endocrine adaptations.

Anatomically, the hypothalamus is bounded anteriorly by the lamina terminalis, posteriorly by the mammillary bodies, inferiorly by the median eminence, and superiorly by the hypothalamic sulcus, which separates it from the thalamus. These boundaries define a compact but highly specialized region whose nuclei are organized into distinct functional zones.

For descriptive clarity, the hypothalamus is divided into three parasagittal zones: the lateral zone, the medial zone, and the periventricular zone. Each contains specific nuclei with specialized physiological roles.

The lateral zone extends throughout the rostrocaudal length of the hypothalamus and contains nuclei involved in arousal, feeding, and sleep regulation. The lateral hypothalamic nucleus has extensive connections with the amygdala and medial prefrontal cortex and is an important center for wakefulness and appetite. It produces orexin, which promotes arousal and stabilizes wakefulness, and melanin-concentrating hormone, which contributes to feeding behavior. Deficiency of orexin is strongly associated with narcolepsy, characterized by sudden and uncontrollable sleep episodes, while reduced melanin-concentrating hormone activity may diminish food intake.

Also within the lateral zone is the lateral preoptic nucleus, which contains sleep-promoting neurons that help initiate and maintain non-rapid eye movement sleep. This nucleus complements the arousal-promoting functions of the lateral hypothalamic region and contributes to the balance between sleep and wakefulness.

The medial zone is functionally the most complex and is subdivided into anterior, middle (tuberal), and posterior (mammillary) regions. These regions contain nuclei that regulate endocrine function, autonomic activity, feeding, temperature, and memory.

The anterior region of the medial zone contains several nuclei essential for thermoregulation, neuroendocrine control, and circadian timing. The anterior nucleus and medial preoptic nucleus are central to heat regulation. They establish the body's thermal set point and mediate heat dissipation through sweating and cutaneous vasodilation. Lesions affecting the anterior hypothalamus may impair heat loss mechanisms and produce hyperthermia.

The medial preoptic nucleus also plays a major neuroendocrine role by secreting gonadotropin-releasing hormone, which stimulates the anterior pituitary to release follicle-stimulating hormone and luteinizing hormone. Through this mechanism, it is essential for reproductive physiology.

The paraventricular nucleus is one of the most important hypothalamic nuclei because of its dual endocrine and autonomic roles. Its magnocellular neurons synthesize oxytocin and vasopressin, which are transported to and released from the posterior pituitary. Its parvocellular neurons produce releasing hormones such as thyrotropin-releasing hormone and corticotropin-releasing hormone, which regulate anterior pituitary function. In addition, a major population of paraventricular neurons projects to autonomic centers in the brainstem and spinal cord, particularly the intermediolateral cell column, forming the Hypothalamospinal pathways. Through these descending projections, the paraventricular nucleus coordinates sympathetic and parasympathetic outflow and links endocrine responses with autonomic control.

The supraoptic nucleus works closely with the paraventricular nucleus and is a major source of vasopressin. Vasopressin promotes renal water reabsorption, supports blood volume, and contributes to vascular tone. Axons from the supraoptic and paraventricular nuclei form the neurohypophysial tract, which terminates in the posterior pituitary. Damage to these nuclei or their axons may result in diabetes insipidus, characterized by excessive urination and thirst due to vasopressin deficiency.

The suprachiasmatic nucleus, located above the optic chiasm in the anterior hypothalamus, functions as the body's master circadian pacemaker. It receives direct photic input from retinal ganglion cells through the retinohypothalamic tract, allowing internal biological rhythms to synchronize with the external light–dark cycle. Through widespread neural projections, the suprachiasmatic nucleus regulates the sleep–wake cycle, melatonin secretion, hormonal rhythms, feeding behavior, metabolism, body temperature, and daily behavioral patterns.

One of the most important outputs of the suprachiasmatic nucleus is the regulation of melatonin synthesis in the pineal gland. This occurs through a multisynaptic pathway extending from the suprachiasmatic nucleus to the paraventricular nucleus, then to the intermediolateral cell column of the spinal cord, onward to the superior cervical ganglion, and finally to the pineal gland. Melatonin reinforces circadian rhythmicity and promotes sleep onset. Lesions of the suprachiasmatic nucleus abolish normal circadian rhythms and may produce sleep disturbances, metabolic dysregulation, mood instability, and cognitive impairment.

The middle, or tuberal, region of the medial zone contains nuclei essential for feeding behavior, energy balance, and endocrine regulation. The dorsomedial nucleus helps regulate feeding, drinking, and body weight. Bilateral lesions may lead to hypophagia and weight loss.

The ventromedial nucleus functions as the principal satiety center. It inhibits feeding behavior and contributes to the regulation of body weight. Lesions of the ventromedial nucleus classically result in hyperphagia, obesity, and sometimes increased irritability or aggressive behavior.

The arcuate nucleus is a major neuroendocrine and metabolic center situated near the median eminence. It secretes several important releasing and inhibitory hormones, including gonadotropin-releasing hormone, growth hormone-releasing hormone, and dopamine, which acts as a prolactin-inhibiting factor. It also plays a central role in appetite regulation through specialized neuronal populations. Neuropeptide Y neurons stimulate feeding, while pro-opiomelanocortin and cocaine- and amphetamine-regulated transcript neurons suppress appetite. Leptin-responsive neurons in the arcuate nucleus signal energy sufficiency and influence both feeding behavior and metabolic rate. Together with the ventromedial nucleus and lateral hypothalamus, the arcuate nucleus forms an integrated network that balances hunger and satiety.

The posterior region of the medial zone includes the posterior nucleus and the mammillary bodies. The posterior nucleus contains cold-sensitive neurons and mediates heat conservation through shivering and peripheral vasoconstriction. Lesions in this region may result in Poikilothermia, in which body temperature varies with the ambient environment because normal thermoregulatory responses are lost.

The mammillary bodies are important components of the limbic system and form part of the Papez circuit. They receive hippocampal input through the fornix and project to the anterior thalamic nucleus via the mammillothalamic tract. Through these pathways, the mammillary bodies contribute to memory processing and emotional integration. Lesions of the mammillary bodies, particularly in chronic thiamine deficiency associated with alcoholism, may produce Korsakoff syndrome, characterized by severe anterograde amnesia, confabulation, and impaired recall.

The periventricular zone lies adjacent to the ependymal lining of the third ventricle and contains smaller neuronal populations involved in neuroendocrine regulation and autonomic modulation. The periventricular nucleus extends through rostral, intermediate, and caudal regions. The rostral part secretes somatostatin and thyrotropin-releasing hormone, the intermediate region produces thyrotropin-releasing hormone, somatostatin, leptin-related signals, gastrin, and neuropeptide Y, while the caudal part contributes to sympathetic regulation. Overall, this zone plays an important role in inhibitory hormonal control and pituitary modulation.

The hypothalamus is the central regulator of body temperature. It maintains the normal thermal set point of approximately 37 degrees Celsius through coordinated actions of several nuclei. Heat-sensitive neurons in the medial preoptic area detect rises in temperature and activate heat-loss mechanisms such as sweating and vasodilation. The anterior hypothalamic region promotes heat dissipation, whereas the posterior hypothalamic region supports heat conservation through shivering and vasoconstriction.

In pyrogenic fever, inflammatory mediators raise the hypothalamic thermal set point through prostaglandin-mediated effects on preoptic neurons. In contrast, in non-pyrogenic hyperthermia such as heat stroke, the set point remains normal, but heat dissipation mechanisms fail. Spinal cord injury may also impair thermoregulation by interrupting descending hypothalamic control over autonomic effectors.

The hypothalamic–pituitary axis is the principal pathway through which the hypothalamus exerts endocrine control. It consists of two major systems: the hypothalamic–neurohypophysial system and the hypothalamic–adenohyphophysial system.

The hypothalamic–neurohypophysial system connects the supraoptic and paraventricular nuclei to the posterior pituitary. Hormones synthesized in these nuclei, mainly oxytocin and vasopressin, are transported down axons through the neurohypophysial tract and stored in nerve terminals in the posterior pituitary. They are then released into the capillary bed for systemic circulation. Oxytocin stimulates uterine contraction and milk ejection, while vasopressin promotes renal water conservation and supports vascular tone. Lesions affecting this pathway may produce diabetes insipidus, whereas excessive vasopressin release can cause the syndrome of inappropriate antidiuretic hormone secretion, leading to water retention and hyponatremia.

The hypothalamic–adenohyphophysial system regulates the anterior pituitary through releasing and inhibitory hormones secreted into the hypophyseal portal circulation. Hormones such as gonadotropin-releasing hormone, growth hormone-releasing hormone, dopamine, thyrotropin-releasing hormone, and corticotropin-releasing hormone are synthesized in nuclei, including the arcuate nucleus, paraventricular nucleus, and medial preoptic region. These hormones enter the primary capillary plexus in the median eminence, supplied by the superior hypophyseal artery, and are carried through the hypophyseal portal veins to the anterior pituitary. There, they regulate the secretion of tropic hormones that control peripheral endocrine glands.

In summary, the hypothalamus is the master regulator of internal homeostasis, integrating neural, autonomic, endocrine, and behavioral responses. Through its highly specialized nuclei and extensive connections, it maintains the stability of the internal environment while allowing the body to adapt dynamically to both internal and external challenges.

Review Questions

Q1. Which hypothalamic nucleus regulates circadian rhythms?
Answer: Suprachiasmatic nucleus (SCN).

Q2. A lesion of the ventromedial nucleus produces what effect?
Answer: Hyperphagia and obesity.

Q3. Which nucleus synthesizes vasopressin?
Answer: Supraoptic nucleus (primary source).

Q4. Orexin deficiency leads to which disorder?
Answer: Narcolepsy.

Q5. Which hypothalamic nucleus is the satiety center?
Answer: Ventromedial nucleus.

Q6. Damage to the mammillary bodies produces which syndrome?
Answer: Korsakoff's amnestic syndrome.

Q7. Which nucleus secretes dopamine to inhibit prolactin?
Answer: Arcuate nucleus.

Q8. Which hypothalamic region mediates heat conservation?
Answer: Posterior nucleus.

Clinical Vignettes

Vignette 1 — Polyuria and Polydipsia
A 45-year-old man develops excessive thirst and passes large volumes of dilute urine after neurosurgery. Serum sodium is elevated.
Most likely damaged nucleus: Supraoptic nucleus → diabetes insipidus.

Vignette 2 — Loss of Circadian Rhythm
A patient with a hypothalamic tumor reports insomnia, daytime sleepiness, and loss of normal sleep–wake cycles.
Affected nucleus: Suprachiasmatic nucleus.

Vignette 3 — Hyperphagia
A 32-year-old woman gains 20 kg over 3 months. MRI shows a lesion in the tuberal hypothalamus.
Damaged nucleus: Ventromedial nucleus.

Vignette 4 — Memory Impairment
A chronic alcoholic presents with confabulation and severe anterograde amnesia.
Affected structure: Mammillary bodies → Korsakoff syndrome.

Vignette 5 — Heat Intolerance
A patient presents with an inability to sweat and persistent hyperthermia after a stroke.
Affected nucleus: Anterior nucleus (heat dissipation center).

Vignette 6 — Narcolepsy
A 19-year-old student experiences sudden daytime sleep episodes.
Deficient neurotransmitter: Orexin (from the lateral hypothalamic nucleus)

Vignette 7 — Prolactin Excess
A woman presents with galactorrhea and amenorrhea. MRI is normal.
Affected nucleus: Arcuate nucleus (dopamine deficiency).

References

1. Gao, Q., & Horvath, T. *Hypothalamus.* In: Encyclopedia of Neuroscience. Springer Nature; 2024.
2. Ocran, E., & Mytilinaios, D. *Hypothalamus: Structure and Functions.* Kenhub; 2023.
3. Dougherty, P. *Hypothalamus: Structural Organization.* Neuroscience Online, McGovern Medical School; 2020.
4. Hoagland, T. M. *Hypothalamus Anatomy: Overview, Gross Anatomy, Microscopic Anatomy.* Medscape; 2025.

Chapter 14

Neurodevelopment and Aging

Click here to view
Chapter Video: https://youtu.be/HIwsufC9xyo

Primary Neurulation and Neural Tube Formation

The earliest visible event in nervous system development is the formation of the neural plate. Around day 18 of embryonic life, inductive signals from the underlying notochord stimulate the overlying ectoderm to thicken and form this specialized neuroectodermal plate. As development proceeds, the neural plate begins to invaginate along its midline, creating a longitudinal depression known as the neural groove. The elevated edges of the groove form the neural folds.

Between days 20 and 22, the neural folds progressively elevate, approach one another, and fuse in the midline to form the neural tube. Fusion begins near the future cervical region and proceeds bidirectionally toward both the cranial and caudal ends. During this period, two temporary openings remain at either end of the tube: the cranial neuropore and the caudal neuropore.

The cranial neuropore normally closes around day 25, whereas the caudal neuropore closes around day 27. Successful closure of these neuropores is essential for normal central nervous system development. Failure of closure results in a spectrum of neural tube defects, many of which are severe or incompatible with life.

Neural Crest Cells: Formation and Migration

During neurulation, a specialized population of cells arises at the crest of the neural folds. These cells undergo epithelial-to-mesenchymal transition and detach from the developing neural tube to form neural crest cells. Neural crest cells are pluripotent and highly migratory, contributing to numerous structures throughout the body.

Within the peripheral nervous system, neural crest cells give rise to dorsal root ganglia, sympathetic chain ganglia, parasympathetic ganglia, and Schwann cells. They also contribute to chromaffin cells of the adrenal medulla, melanocytes, craniofacial bones and cartilage, odontoblasts, and the conotruncal septum of the developing heart.

The broad developmental potential of neural crest cells explains the diverse clinical manifestations associated with defects in their migration or differentiation. Hirschsprung disease results from the failed migration of enteric neural crest cells, producing aganglionic megacolon. Waardenburg syndrome is characterized by pigmentary abnormalities and sensorineural deafness due to abnormal neural crest derivatives. DiGeorge syndrome involves defective neural crest development, contributing to conotruncal cardiac malformations and thymic hypoplasia.

Regionalization of the Neural Tube

Following closure, the neural tube undergoes rapid regional specialization. The cranial two-thirds expand and differentiate to form the brain, whereas the caudal one-third develops into the spinal cord. The central lumen of the neural tube persists throughout development and gives rise to the ventricular system and central canal. This early regionalization establishes the basic structural framework for future central nervous system organization and compartmentalization.

Neural Tube Defects

Failure of normal neural tube closure results in characteristic congenital malformations. Failure of closure of the cranial neuropore results in anencephaly, a severe defect characterized by the absence of the calvarium and much of the cerebral hemispheres. Defective cranial closure may also produce a meningoencephalocele, in which meninges and brain tissue herniate through a skull defect.

Defects of caudal neuropore closure produce the various forms of spina bifida. In spina bifida occulta, there is failure of vertebral arch fusion without herniation of neural tissue, often presenting clinically with a tuft of hair or cutaneous dimple. Meningocele involves the herniation of meninges through a vertebral defect, whereas myelomeningocele is a more severe lesion in which both meninges and spinal cord tissue protrude. Craniorachischisis represents complete failure of neural tube closure along the craniospinal axis and is incompatible with life.

Prenatal screening plays an important role in the early detection of open neural tube defects. Maternal serum alpha-fetoprotein levels and amniotic fluid acetylcholinesterase are typically elevated in open defects. Prenatal ultrasonography provides definitive anatomical confirmation and helps guide clinical management.

Formation of the Brain Vesicles

As the cranial neural tube enlarges, it forms three primary brain vesicles: the prosencephalon, mesencephalon, and rhombencephalon. These primitive vesicles represent the earliest subdivisions of the developing brain. Simultaneously, the cephalic and cervical flexures develop, creating the characteristic curvature of the embryonic neural axis.

By the fifth week of development, the primary vesicles differentiate into five secondary brain vesicles. The prosencephalon divides into the telencephalon and diencephalon. The telencephalon gives rise to the cerebral hemispheres, basal ganglia, and limbic structures, while the diencephalon forms the thalamus, hypothalamus, retina, and pineal gland. The associated ventricular cavity develops into the lateral ventricles and the third ventricle. The mesencephalon remains undivided and develops into the midbrain, including the tectum, tegmentum, and substantia nigra. Its cavity persists as the cerebral aqueduct. The rhombencephalon divides into the metencephalon and myelencephalon. The metencephalon gives rise to the pons and cerebellum, while the myelencephalon forms the medulla oblongata. These structures are associated with the fourth ventricle. This vesicular organization provides the basic blueprint for mature brain architecture.

Cortical Expansion and Gyrification

The telencephalon undergoes rapid growth during fetal development, resulting in the formation of the bilateral cerebral hemispheres. As the cerebral cortex expands, its surface area increases dramatically through the formation of gyri and sulci, a process known as gyrification.

Gyrification occurs most prominently between 24 and 34 weeks of gestation. This process allows a greater number of neurons and synaptic connections to be accommodated within the limited confines of the cranial vault, thereby enhancing cognitive capacity and functional complexity.

Development of the Meninges

The meninges develop from both neural crest and mesodermal tissues, reflecting the close interaction between neural and mesenchymal embryologic structures. The pia mater and arachnoid mater, collectively known as the leptomeninges, are derived primarily from neural crest cells. In contrast, the dura mater, or pachymeninx, develops mainly from mesoderm. This dual embryologic origin is important in understanding congenital meningeal malformations and the developmental relationships between the coverings of the central nervous system and adjacent craniofacial structures.

Development of the Ventricular System

The ventricular system arises directly from the lumen of the embryonic neural tube. As the telencephalon expands, paired lateral ventricles develop within the cerebral hemispheres. These communicate with the third ventricle through the interventricular foramina of Monro. The third ventricle connects to the fourth ventricle through the cerebral aqueduct, which traverses the midbrain. The fourth ventricle is continuous caudally with the central canal of the spinal cord. Normal cerebrospinal fluid circulation depends on the patency of this ventricular system. Obstruction at any point in the pathway may result in hydrocephalus, with potentially significant effects on brain development and function.

Understanding early nervous system development is essential not only for appreciating the structural complexity of the adult brain and spinal cord but also for recognizing the embryologic basis of many neurologic and congenital disorders.

Postnatal Brain Development and Aging

Postnatal brain development is a prolonged and highly dynamic process that extends from late fetal life into early adulthood. It is characterized by progressive myelination, synaptic remodeling, and the maturation of functional neural systems that underlie cognition and behavior.

Myelination begins prenatally but continues well into the third decade of life, reflecting the gradual optimization of neural transmission. The sequence of myelination follows a functional hierarchy: primary sensory pathways myelinate early, enabling basic perception soon after birth, whereas higher-order association areas, particularly the prefrontal cortex, are among the last regions to mature. This delayed maturation underlies the prolonged development of executive functions such as planning, decision-making, and impulse control.

Another critical feature of postnatal development is synaptic pruning, a process that peaks during childhood and adolescence. During this period, excess synaptic connections formed earlier in development are selectively eliminated, while frequently used synapses are strengthened. This activity-dependent refinement enhances the efficiency and specificity of neural circuits, allowing the brain to adapt to environmental demands.

The concept of critical periods is central to understanding early brain development. These are time windows during which specific neural systems are particularly sensitive to environmental input. Functions such as vision, language acquisition, and social bonding depend heavily on appropriate stimulation during these periods. Deprivation or abnormal experience during critical periods can lead to long-lasting deficits that are difficult to reverse later in life.

The maturation of cognitive and behavioral systems follows a predictable sequence. Sensory systems develop early, providing the foundation for interaction with the environment. Motor development is closely linked to the myelination of descending pathways, particularly the corticospinal tract, which supports the acquisition of motor milestones. Language networks undergo progressive specialization, with left hemispheric dominance typically established by 5 to 7 years of age. In contrast, executive functions continue to mature into early adulthood, paralleling the prolonged development of the prefrontal cortex.

Neural plasticity, the capacity of the brain to reorganize structurally and functionally, varies across the lifespan. In childhood, plasticity is at its peak, allowing remarkable recovery from injury and adaptability to new experiences. In adulthood, plasticity persists but is more limited, forming the basis for learning and rehabilitation following neurological damage. With aging, plasticity gradually declines; however, the concept of cognitive reserve—built through education, intellectual engagement, and life experiences—can buffer against functional deterioration.

Aging of the nervous system is associated with both structural and functional changes. Structurally, there is progressive cortical thinning, hippocampal atrophy, loss of white matter integrity, and a reduction in synaptic density. These changes contribute to the decline in neural efficiency observed in older individuals. Functionally, aging is characterized by a slowing of information processing, along with declines in working memory and executive function. In contrast, certain cognitive domains, such as semantic memory and vocabulary, are relatively preserved, reflecting the stability of well-established knowledge networks.

Neurochemical alterations also play a significant role in age-related changes. Dopaminergic activity declines with age, contributing to slowed motor function and reduced motivation. Cholinergic deficits are associated with impairments in memory and attention, while alterations in serotonin and norepinephrine systems

Summary of Development

- Neural tube → CNS; neural crest → PNS
- Myelination continues into adulthood
- Synaptic pruning enhances efficiency
- Critical periods shape sensory/language development

Plasticity

- High in childhood
- Present in adulthood
- Declines with aging

Development of Cognitive and Behavioral Systems

- Sensory systems mature early
- Motor systems → corticospinal tract myelination supports milestones
- Language networks → left hemisphere specialization by age 5–7
- Executive function → prefrontal cortex matures into early adulthood

Aging of the Nervous System

Structural Changes

- Cortical thinning
- Hippocampal atrophy
- White matter loss
- Reduced synaptic density

Functional Changes

- Slowed processing speed
- Decline in working memory and executive function
- Preserved semantic memory and vocabulary

Neurochemical Changes

- Reduced dopamine → slowed movement, reduced motivation
- Reduced acetylcholine → memory impairment
- Altered serotonin and norepinephrine → mood changes

Neurodegenerative Diseases

- Alzheimer's disease → hippocampal atrophy, amyloid plaques, tau tangles
- Parkinson's disease → dopaminergic loss in substantia nigra, bradykinesia, tremor
- Frontotemporal dementia → behavioral/language changes, frontal/temporal atrophy
- Vascular cognitive impairment → smallvessel disease, executive dysfunction
- Alzheimer's, Parkinson's, FTD, vascular dementia

Review Questions

Q1. Which cortical region matures last?
Answer: Prefrontal cortex.

Q2. What embryological defect causes lissencephaly?
Answer: Impaired neuronal migration.

Q3. What process refines circuits during adolescence?
Answer: Synaptic pruning.

Q4. Which neurotransmitter declines with aging, impairing memory?
Answer: Acetylcholine.

Q5. What structure is affected early in Alzheimer's disease?
Answer: Hippocampus.

Clinical Vignettes

Vignette 1 — Developmental Delay
Delayed motor milestones and hypotonia.
Localization: Delayed corticospinal tract myelination.

Vignette 2 — Early Alzheimer's Disease
Progressive memory impairment in a 68-year-old.
Localization: Hippocampal degeneration.

Vignette 3 — Autism Spectrum Disorder
Impaired social reciprocity and restricted interests.
Localization: Altered connectivity in social cognition networks.

Vignette 4 — Stroke Recovery
Functional improvement months after stroke.
Mechanism: Adult neuroplasticity.

Reference

1. Kandel ER, Schwartz JH, Jessell TM, Siegelbaum SA, Hudspeth AJ. *Principles of Neural Science*. 5th ed. McGraw-Hill; 2013.
2. Purves D, Augustine GJ, Fitzpatrick D, et al. *Neuroscience*. 6th ed. Oxford University Press; 2018.
3. Schmahmann JD. *The cerebellar cognitive affective syndrome and the cerebellum's role in cognition*. Brain. 1998;121(4):561579.
4. Morrison JH, Hof PR. *Life and death of neurons in the aging brain*. Science. 1997;278(5337):412419.

Chapter 15

Arterial Supply of the Brain: Internal Carotid System, Vertebrobasilar System, and Major Cerebral Arteries

Click here to view
Chapter Video: https://youtu.be/0jgKAAHOOl0

The arterial supply of the brain is derived from two major paired systems: the internal carotid arteries and the vertebral arteries. These vessels ascend through the neck, enter the cranial cavity, and anastomose on the inferior surface of the brain to form the arterial circle known as the Circle of Willis. This anastomotic ring provides an important mechanism for collateral circulation, allowing partial compensation when one component of the cerebral circulation is compromised. From this circle arise the principal cerebral arteries—the anterior, middle, and posterior cerebral arteries—which distribute blood to the cerebral hemispheres and deep brain structures.

The brain has an exceptionally high metabolic demand and minimal energy reserves. Consequently, interruption of cerebral blood flow for even a few minutes can result in irreversible neuronal injury. A detailed understanding of the arterial supply is therefore essential for interpreting cerebrovascular disease and accurately localizing neurological deficits.

The internal carotid artery system constitutes the anterior circulation of the brain. Each internal carotid artery enters the cranial cavity through the carotid canal, traverses the cavernous sinus, and forms a characteristic S-shaped curve known as the carotid siphon. After piercing the dura to enter the subarachnoid space, it gives rise to several important branches before terminating by dividing into the anterior cerebral artery and the middle cerebral artery. Among its branches, the posterior communicating artery is particularly significant, as it connects the internal carotid system with the posterior cerebral artery and contributes to the Circle of Willis.

The anterior cerebral artery courses anteriorly and superiorly within the interhemispheric fissure, closely following the curvature of the corpus callosum. The two anterior cerebral arteries are interconnected by the anterior communicating artery, completing the anterior portion of the Circle of Willis. The anterior cerebral artery supplies the medial surfaces of the frontal and parietal lobes, including the superior frontal gyrus and the paracentral lobule, which contains the cortical representation of the contralateral lower limb. It also supplies the rostrum, genu, and body of the corpus callosum.

Occlusion of the anterior cerebral artery produces a characteristic clinical syndrome dominated by contralateral weakness and sensory loss in the lower limb. Because of the involvement of medial frontal regions, urinary incontinence may occur due to impairment of higher control over micturition. Involvement of the supplementary motor area can lead to apraxia, particularly when the dominant hemisphere is affected. Damage to the corpus callosum may result in disconnection syndromes, reflecting impaired interhemispheric communication.

The middle cerebral artery is the largest branch of the internal carotid artery and the vessel most commonly involved in ischemic stroke. It passes laterally into the lateral sulcus and divides into a series of segments that supply both cortical and deep structures. Its cortical branches supply nearly the entire lateral surface of the cerebral hemisphere, including the primary motor and sensory cortices for the face and upper limb, language areas such as Broca's and Wernicke's areas in the dominant hemisphere, the frontal eye field, the inferior parietal lobule, and the primary auditory cortex.

In addition to its cortical branches, the middle cerebral artery gives rise to small but clinically crucial perforating vessels known as the lenticulostriate arteries. These vessels supply the basal ganglia and the internal capsule, particularly the posterior limb. Because of their small caliber and susceptibility to pathological changes such as lipohyalinosis, they are a common site of lacunar infarcts.

Occlusion of the middle cerebral artery produces a range of neurological deficits depending on whether the dominant or non-dominant hemisphere is involved. In the dominant hemisphere, infarction typically results in contralateral weakness and sensory loss affecting the face and upper limb, along with aphasia due to involvement of language areas. In the non-dominant hemisphere, similar motor and sensory deficits occur, but are accompanied by hemispatial neglect, particularly of the contralateral side. Visual field defects, such as homonymous hemianopia, are common due to involvement of the optic radiations. Lacunar infarcts involving the lenticulostriate arteries produce characteristic syndromes such as pure motor stroke, pure sensory stroke, ataxic hemiparesis, and dysarthria–clumsy hand syndrome, typically without cortical signs such as aphasia or neglect.

The vertebrobasilar system constitutes the posterior circulation of the brain. The vertebral arteries enter the cranial cavity through the foramen magnum and ascend along the ventral surface of the medulla. At the level of the lower border of the pons, they unite to form the basilar artery. The basilar artery ascends along the ventral surface of the pons and ultimately bifurcates into the posterior cerebral arteries.

The posterior cerebral artery supplies the occipital lobe, including the primary and association visual cortices, as well as the inferior and medial aspects of the temporal lobe. It also supplies important deep structures, including the hippocampus, amygdala, posterior thalamus, geniculate bodies, and the splenium of the corpus callosum. Through its posterior choroidal branches, it contributes to the vascular supply of the dorsal thalamus, pineal gland, and choroid plexus of the third ventricle.

Occlusion of the posterior cerebral artery most commonly produces contralateral homonymous hemianopia, often with macular sparing due to collateral supply from the middle cerebral artery. Involvement of the thalamus may result in contralateral hemisensory loss and the development of central post-stroke pain, known as thalamic pain syndrome or Dejerine–Roussy syndrome. Damage to the hippocampus can produce memory deficits, particularly anterograde amnesia. Lesions involving the visual association cortex may lead to higher-order visual disturbances such as visual agnosia, achromatopsia, and prosopagnosia. Involvement of the splenium of the corpus callosum may produce alexia without agraphia, a distinctive disconnection syndrome in which the patient cannot read but can still write.

Compromise of the vertebrobasilar circulation may produce a constellation of symptoms referred to as vertebrobasilar insufficiency. Because this system supplies the brainstem, cerebellum, occipital lobes, and parts of the thalamus, the clinical presentation is often complex and multifocal. Patients may experience vertigo, diplopia, visual disturbances, dysarthria, ataxia, sudden falls known as drop attacks, and transient sensory symptoms. These manifestations reflect transient ischemia of structures critical for balance, coordination, vision, and cranial nerve function.

In addition to territory-specific infarcts, the brain is also susceptible to watershed infarctions. These occur in border zone regions between the major cerebral arteries and are particularly vulnerable to systemic hypotension or global hypoperfusion. The watershed zone between the anterior and middle cerebral arteries typically involves regions controlling proximal limb function, and bilateral involvement may produce the characteristic "man in the barrel" syndrome, in which arm weakness is more pronounced than leg weakness. The watershed region between the middle and posterior cerebral arteries is associated with higher-order visual and cognitive functions, and infarction in this area may result in visual processing deficits and memory impairment.

In summary, the arterial supply of the brain is organized into anterior and posterior circulatory systems that converge at the Circle of Willis. The anterior cerebral, middle cerebral, and posterior cerebral arteries supply distinct but functionally interrelated territories. Knowledge of these vascular distributions, along with their clinical correlates, provides a critical foundation for understanding stroke syndromes, guiding diagnosis, and informing therapeutic strategies in cerebrovascular disease.

Review Questions

Q1. Which artery supplies the paracentral lobule?
Answer: Anterior cerebral artery (ACA).

Q2. Which vessel is most commonly involved in ischemic stroke?
Answer: Middle cerebral artery (MCA).

Q3. What is the hallmark of a PCA stroke?
Answer: Contralateral homonymous hemianopia with macular sparing.

Q4. Which arteries supply the internal capsule?
Answer: Lenticulostriate arteries (MCA) and the anterior choroidal artery.

Q5. What syndrome results from splenial infarction?
Answer: Alexia without agraphia.

Clinical Vignette

A 58-year-old man with hypertension develops right facial droop, right arm weakness, and difficulty speaking. His eyes deviate to the left. He cannot repeat phrases but understands simple commands. Sensation is intact. MRI shows an infarct in the left inferior frontal gyrus and adjacent insular cortex.

Diagnosis: Left dominant MCA stroke involving Broca's area.
Explanation: The MCA supplies the lateral frontal lobe, including the motor cortex for face and arm, and the dominanthemisphere language areas. Conjugate gaze deviation toward the lesion reflects frontal eye field involvement.

References

1. Standring, S. (Ed.) *Gray's Anatomy: The Anatomical Basis of Clinical Practice*. Elsevier.
   Definitive anatomical descriptions of cerebral arteries, Circle of Willis, and vascular territories.
2. Haines, D. E. *Neuroanatomy: An Atlas of Structures, Sections, and Systems*. Wolters Kluwer.
   Clear vascular maps, internal capsule supply, and brainstem circulation.
3. Caplan, L. R. *Caplan's Stroke: A Clinical Approach*. Cambridge University Press.
   Authoritative coverage of stroke syndromes, lacunar infarcts, and vertebrobasilar disease.
4. Mohr, J. P., Wolf, P. A., et al. *Stroke: Pathophysiology, Diagnosis, and Management*. Elsevier.
   Comprehensive review of anterior and posterior circulation strokes and watershed infarcts.
5. Rhoton, A. L. *Cranial Anatomy and Surgical Approaches*. Neurosurgery Supplement.
   Detailed microanatomy of cerebral arteries, perforators, and deep vascular territories.

Chapter 16

Stroke Mechanism: Neuroanatomy and Pathophysiology

Click here to view
Chapter Video: https://youtu.be/hi8slkuvBWY

Stroke is one of the most clinically significant disorders of the nervous system and remains a leading cause of mortality and long-term disability worldwide. It is characterized by the sudden onset of a focal neurological deficit resulting from interruption of cerebral blood flow. The defining feature of stroke is its abrupt presentation, reflecting the acute nature of vascular compromise rather than a gradual pathological process. Because the brain has minimal energy reserves and depends on continuous perfusion, even brief interruptions in blood supply can produce rapid and irreversible neuronal injury.

Broadly, stroke syndromes arise from two fundamental mechanisms: ischemia and hemorrhage. Ischemic stroke results from obstruction of blood flow due to thrombosis, embolism, or systemic hypoperfusion, whereas hemorrhagic stroke occurs when a blood vessel ruptures, leading to extravasation of blood into or around the brain. A closely related clinical entity is the transient ischemic attack, which represents a temporary disruption of cerebral perfusion without permanent tissue injury.

A transient ischemic attack is defined as a brief episode of neurological dysfunction caused by transient cerebral ischemia. By definition, symptoms resolve completely, typically within minutes and always within twenty-four hours, and there is no evidence of infarction on neuroimaging. Despite its transient nature, a transient ischemic attack is of great clinical importance, as it serves as a warning sign of impending stroke. The risk of progression to a completed infarction is highest within the first forty-eight hours, and a significant proportion of patients will develop a stroke within the following weeks if appropriate intervention is not undertaken. For this reason, transient ischemic attacks demand urgent evaluation and aggressive risk factor management.

Ischemic stroke accounts for the vast majority of cases, comprising approximately eighty-five percent of all strokes. It most commonly results from thrombotic occlusion of a cerebral artery, embolic obstruction originating from the heart or large vessels, or global reduction in cerebral perfusion. The underlying pathophysiological process is known as the ischemic cascade, a sequence of biochemical and cellular events triggered by inadequate blood flow.

Within minutes of ischemia, depletion of adenosine triphosphate leads to failure of energy-dependent ion pumps, particularly the sodium–potassium ATPase. This results in intracellular accumulation of sodium and water, producing cytotoxic edema. Simultaneously, there is excessive release of excitatory neurotransmitters, particularly glutamate, which overstimulates postsynaptic receptors and leads to calcium influx. Elevated intracellular calcium activates a range of destructive enzymes, including proteases, lipases, and endonucleases, which degrade cellular structures. Mitochondrial dysfunction ensues, leading to the generation of free radicals and further cellular injury. Ultimately, these processes culminate in neuronal death through both necrosis and apoptosis.

Within the ischemic region, two zones can be identified. The central core represents tissue that has suffered irreversible damage due to critically reduced blood flow. Surrounding this is the ischemic penumbra, a region of functionally impaired but potentially viable tissue. The penumbra is the primary target of acute therapeutic interventions, as timely restoration of perfusion can salvage this tissue and improve clinical outcomes.

Hemorrhagic stroke, in contrast, results from rupture of intracranial vessels and accounts for a smaller but often more severe proportion of strokes. It includes intracerebral hemorrhage, in which bleeding occurs within the brain parenchyma, and subarachnoid hemorrhage, in which blood accumulates in the subarachnoid space. The mechanisms of injury in hemorrhagic stroke differ from those in ischemia and include direct mechanical damage from the expanding hematoma, increased intracranial pressure, reduced cerebral perfusion due to mass effect, and toxic effects of blood breakdown products on neural tissue. Common etiological factors include chronic hypertension, rupture of saccular aneurysms, arteriovenous malformations, and cerebral amyloid angiopathy.

Several risk factors contribute to the development of stroke. Among these, hypertension is the most significant modifiable factor, exerting a major influence on both ischemic and hemorrhagic stroke risk. Other modifiable factors include diabetes mellitus, Hyperlipidemia, smoking, atrial fibrillation, carotid artery disease, obesity, sedentary lifestyle, and excessive alcohol consumption. Non-modifiable risk factors include advancing age, genetic predisposition, and a prior history of stroke or transient ischemic attack.

The early management of stroke is directed toward rapid recognition, prompt diagnosis, and timely intervention to limit neuronal injury. Immediate neuroimaging, typically with computed tomography or magnetic resonance imaging, is essential to distinguish between ischemic and hemorrhagic stroke, as the management strategies differ fundamentally. In ischemic stroke, reperfusion therapy is the cornerstone of treatment. Intravenous thrombolysis with tissue plasminogen activator, administered within the appropriate therapeutic window, can restore blood flow and salvage the ischemic penumbra. In selected cases of large vessel occlusion, mechanical thrombectomy offers an effective means of revascularization. Supportive measures, including control of blood pressure, glucose, temperature, and oxygenation, are critical in optimizing outcomes. In patients with atrial fibrillation, anticoagulation is essential to prevent recurrent embolic events, while antiplatelet therapy is indicated in other forms of ischemic stroke. The principle that "time is brain" underscores the urgency of these interventions.

Stroke syndromes reflect the specific vascular territory involved and provide important clues for anatomical localization. Occlusion of the anterior cerebral artery typically produces weakness and sensory loss predominantly affecting the contralateral lower limb. Middle cerebral artery infarction results in deficits involving the face and upper limb, often accompanied by aphasia in the dominant hemisphere or hemispatial neglect in the non-dominant hemisphere. Posterior cerebral artery stroke primarily affects visual pathways, leading to contralateral homonymous hemianopia and, in some cases, higher-order visual disturbances. Lacunar infarcts, resulting from occlusion of small penetrating arteries, produce characteristic syndromes such as pure motor or pure sensory deficits without cortical signs.

In summary, stroke represents an acute disruption of cerebral function due to vascular compromise. Its pathophysiology involves complex interactions between vascular, metabolic, and cellular mechanisms, leading to rapid neuronal injury. A clear understanding of these processes, along with the vascular anatomy of the brain, is essential for accurate diagnosis, effective management, and prevention of this major neurological disorder.

A stroke syndrome refers to the constellation of neurological deficits arising from the interruption of blood flow to a specific vascular territory.

Because each artery supplies distinct regions, the pattern of deficits helps localize the lesion.

Examples

- ACA stroke → leg weakness
- MCA stroke → face/arm weakness, aphasia, neglect
- PCA stroke → visual field deficits
- Lacunar stroke → pure motor or pure sensory deficits

Review Questions

Q1. What distinguishes a TIA from an ischemic stroke?
Answer: Symptoms resolve within 24 hours, and no infarction is seen on imaging.

Q2. What is the most important modifiable risk factor for stroke?
Answer: Hypertension.

Q3. What is the ischemic penumbra?
Answer: Viable but at-risk tissue surrounding the core infarct.

Q4. What is the primary mechanism of neuronal injury in ischemic stroke?
Answer: Excitotoxicity due to glutamate release and calcium influx.

Q5. What is the hallmark of hemorrhagic stroke?
Answer: Extravasation of blood into the brain parenchyma or subarachnoid space.

Clinical Vignette

A 67-year-old man with hypertension and atrial fibrillation experiences sudden rightsided weakness and difficulty speaking. Symptoms resolve completely within 45 minutes. MRI shows no infarction.

Diagnosis: Transient ischemic attack (TIA).
Explanation: The sudden onset, rapid resolution, and absence of imaging abnormalities are characteristic of TIA. His atrial fibrillation places him at high risk for embolic stroke, and early anticoagulation is essential to prevent progression to a frank infarct.

Reference

1. Kandel ER, Schwartz JH, Jessell TM, Siegelbaum SA, Hudspeth AJ. *Principles of Neural Science*. 5th ed. McGraw-Hill; 2013.
2. Purves D, Augustine GJ, Fitzpatrick D, et al. *Neuroscience*. 6th ed. Oxford University Press; 2018.
3. Neuroanatomy Through Clinical Cases
   Blumenfeld H. *Neuroanatomy Through Clinical Cases*. 3rd ed. Sinauer Associates.

Chapter 17

Brainstem Stroke Pattern Neuroanatomy, Vascular Syndromes, and Clinical Correlates

Click here to view
Chapter Video: https://youtu.be/FSF_S_1d09c

A brainstem stroke refers to an infarction or hemorrhage involving the midbrain, pons, or medulla. Although the brainstem is relatively small in size, it contains a dense concentration of vital neural structures, including ascending sensory pathways, descending motor tracts, cranial nerve nuclei, and autonomic centers responsible for respiration and cardiovascular regulation. Consequently, even a small lesion in this region can produce profound and potentially life-threatening neurological deficits.

Brainstem strokes arise from a variety of vascular mechanisms. Small vessel disease, particularly lipohyalinosis affecting penetrating arteries, is a common cause of focal lesions. Larger vessel pathology, including atherosclerosis of the vertebral or basilar arteries, may lead to more extensive infarction. Thromboembolism and intracranial hemorrhage also contribute to brainstem stroke syndromes. The clinical presentation is highly variable, ranging from isolated cranial nerve deficits to catastrophic impairment of consciousness, breathing, and circulatory control. Accurate diagnosis and localization require a thorough understanding of brainstem neuroanatomy and vascular supply.

The organization of cranial nerve nuclei within the brainstem follows a consistent rostrocaudal pattern that provides a useful framework for clinical localization. In the midbrain are the nuclei of the oculomotor and trochlear nerves. The pons contains the nuclei of the trigeminal, abducens, facial, and vestibulocochlear nerves. The medulla houses the nuclei of the glossopharyngeal, vagus, cranial component of the accessory nerve, and hypoglossal nerve. This orderly arrangement allows clinicians to correlate specific cranial nerve deficits with the level of the lesion.

Functionally, the brainstem can also be divided into medial (paramedian) and lateral regions. The paramedian region primarily contains motor structures, including descending corticospinal fibers, the medial lemniscus, the medial longitudinal fasciculus, and motor cranial nerve nuclei such as those of the oculomotor, trochlear, abducens, and hypoglossal nerves. In contrast, the lateral region contains mixed sensory and motor nuclei, including those associated with the trigeminal, facial, glossopharyngeal, and vagus nerves, as well as purely sensory nuclei such as the vestibular and cochlear nuclei. This anatomical arrangement underlies the characteristic patterns of deficits seen in brainstem stroke.

Lesions affecting the paramedian region typically involve the corticospinal tract, resulting in contralateral weakness or hemiplegia. Involvement of the medial lemniscus produces contralateral loss of fine touch, vibration, and proprioception. Damage to the medial longitudinal fasciculus leads to internuclear ophthalmoplegia, characterized by failure of adduction of the ipsilateral eye and nystagmus of the contralateral abducting eye. Because the motor cranial nerve nuclei are located in this region, lesions produce ipsilateral cranial nerve palsies. The combination of ipsilateral cranial nerve deficits with contralateral motor or sensory deficits gives rise to the classic "crossed findings" that are a hallmark of brainstem lesions.

Medial brainstem syndromes are defined by these characteristic patterns. In medial medullary syndrome, which results from occlusion of the anterior spinal artery, patients exhibit contralateral weakness due to corticospinal tract involvement, contralateral loss of proprioception and vibration from medial lemniscus damage, and ipsilateral deviation of the tongue due to involvement of the hypoglossal nerve. In medial pontine syndrome, caused by occlusion of paramedian branches of the basilar artery, similar findings are present, including contralateral hemiparesis and sensory loss, accompanied by ipsilateral abducens nerve palsy, resulting in impaired lateral gaze.

In contrast, **lateral brainstem syndromes** involve structures such as the spinothalamic tract, spinocerebellar pathways, spinal trigeminal tract, and descending sympathetic fibers. Damage to the spinothalamic tract produces contralateral loss of pain and temperature sensation from the body, while involvement of the spinal trigeminal tract causes ipsilateral loss of pain and temperature sensation from the face. Lesions of the spinocerebellar pathways result in ipsilateral ataxia, and disruption of descending sympathetic fibers leads to ipsilateral Horner syndrome, characterized by ptosis, miosis, and anhidrosis.

The prototypical lateral brainstem syndrome is lateral medullary syndrome, also known as **Wallenberg syndrome**, most commonly caused by occlusion of the posterior inferior cerebellar artery. This condition affects the dorsolateral medulla and produces a distinctive constellation of findings. Patients develop ipsilateral facial pain and temperature loss along with contralateral loss of pain and temperature sensation in the body, reflecting involvement of the spinal trigeminal and spinothalamic tracts. Dysphagia and hoarseness occur due to involvement of the nucleus ambiguus, which supplies the glossopharyngeal and vagus nerves. Vestibular nuclei involvement leads to vertigo and nystagmus, while damage to the inferior cerebellar peduncle causes ipsilateral ataxia. Ipsilateral Horner syndrome results from the disruption of sympathetic pathways. The involvement of the nucleus ambiguus is a key distinguishing feature of posterior inferior cerebellar artery infarction.

Large vessel occlusion within the vertebrobasilar system can produce devastating neurological consequences. Occlusion of the basilar artery, in particular, may result in quadriplegia and the so-called locked-in syndrome, in which the patient is conscious but unable to move or speak due to paralysis of nearly all voluntary muscles except for vertical eye movements. Involvement of the reticular activating system may lead to coma, while disruption of autonomic centers can cause respiratory failure and cardiovascular instability. These conditions represent neurological emergencies requiring immediate recognition and intervention.

Advances in neuroimaging have significantly improved the diagnosis and management of brainstem stroke. High-resolution magnetic resonance imaging can detect small infarcts that were previously difficult to visualize. Perfusion imaging techniques allow identification of ischemic but potentially salvageable tissue within the posterior circulation. In selected cases, mechanical thrombectomy has emerged as an effective treatment for basilar artery occlusion, improving outcomes in what was once considered a uniformly fatal condition.

In summary, brainstem stroke represents a unique and often severe form of cerebrovascular disease characterized by complex neurological deficits. The precise pattern of clinical findings reflects the highly organized anatomy of the brainstem, with distinct medial and lateral syndromes corresponding to specific vascular territories. A thorough understanding of these anatomical and functional relationships is essential for accurate localization, prompt diagnosis, and effective management of these potentially life-threatening conditions.

Review Questions

Q1. Which artery is most commonly occluded in lateral medullary syndrome?
Posterior inferior cerebellar artery (PICA).

Q2. What is the hallmark of medial medullary syndrome?
Contralateral hemiparesis + contralateral proprioception loss + ipsilateral tongue deviation.

Q3. Which cranial nerve palsy is characteristic of a paramedian pontine infarct?
CN VI palsy.

Q4. What structure is damaged in internuclear ophthalmoplegia?
Medial longitudinal fasciculus (MLF).

Q5. What is the classic pattern of crossed findings in brainstem stroke?
Ipsilateral cranial nerve deficit with contralateral body weakness.

Clinical Vignette

A 63-year-old man presents with sudden vertigo, hoarseness, dysphagia, and loss of pain sensation on the right side of his face. He also has loss of pain and temperature on the left side of his body and right-sided Horner syndrome.

Diagnosis: Right-sided lateral medullary (Wallenberg) syndrome.
Explanation: The combination of nucleus ambiguus dysfunction, ipsilateral facial sensory loss, contralateral body sensory loss, and Horner syndrome localizes the lesion to the dorsolateral medulla, typically due to PICA occlusion.

References

1. Kandel, E. R., Schwartz, J. H., Jessell, T. M., et al. *Principles of Neural Science*. McGraw-Hill.
   Foundational coverage of brainstem anatomy, cranial nerve nuclei, and vascular territories.
2. Haines, D. E. *Neuroanatomy: An Atlas of Structures, Sections, and Systems*. Wolters Kluwer.
   Detailed structural maps of the midbrain, pons, and medulla with vascular overlays.
3. Caplan, L. R. *Caplan's Stroke: A Clinical Approach*. Cambridge University Press.
   Authoritative descriptions of vertebrobasilar syndromes, Wallenberg syndrome, and basilar artery occlusion.

4. Rhoton, A. L. *Cranial Anatomy and Surgical Approaches.* Neurosurgery Supplement.
High-resolution microanatomy of brainstem vasculature and perforating arteries.

5. Fisher, C. M. "Lacunar Strokes and Brainstem Syndromes." *Neurology.*
Classic clinical–pathological correlations for paramedian and lateral brainstem infarcts.

Chapter 18

Blood-Brain Barrier: Neurovascular Principles Structure, Function, Clinical Correlates

---

Click here to view
Chapter Video: https://youtu.be/SIVXWIrk0yk

The blood–brain barrier is a highly specialized interface that separates the systemic circulation from the central nervous system. It plays a crucial role in maintaining the stability of the neural microenvironment by protecting brain tissue from potentially harmful substances while allowing the selective entry of essential nutrients, ions, and signaling molecules. As a fundamental component of neurovascular physiology, it influences not only homeostasis but also drug delivery, immune interactions, and the pathogenesis of neurological disease.

Structurally, the blood–brain barrier is formed primarily by the endothelial cells lining cerebral capillaries. Unlike peripheral capillaries, these endothelial cells are non-fenestrated and are tightly sealed by complex junctional proteins, including claudins, occludins, and zonula occludens proteins. These tight junctions effectively eliminate paracellular transport, forcing substances to pass through the cells rather than between them. Surrounding the endothelial layer is a basement membrane that provides structural support and contributes to barrier integrity.

Embedded within this vascular framework are pericytes, which play an important role in regulating capillary blood flow, maintaining vascular stability, and contributing to angiogenesis. Enveloping the capillaries are the astrocytic end feet, which form a nearly continuous sheath around the vessels. Astrocytes secrete factors that are essential for the development and maintenance of the barrier properties of endothelial cells, thereby reinforcing the functional integrity of the blood–brain barrier.

Transport across the blood–brain barrier is highly selective and tightly regulated. Essential nutrients such as glucose are transported via specific carrier systems, notably the GLUT1 transporter, while amino acids and ions are conveyed through specialized channels and transporters. At the same time, efflux systems, including P-glycoprotein and other ATP-dependent transporters, actively remove potentially harmful substances and many pharmacological agents from the brain, thereby limiting their accumulation.

The blood–brain barrier is not an isolated structure, but forms part of a broader functional entity known as the neurovascular unit. This unit includes endothelial cells, pericytes, astrocytes, neurons, and microglia, all of which interact dynamically to regulate cerebral blood flow in response to neuronal activity. This process, termed neurovascular coupling, ensures that regions of increased neuronal activity receive an adequate supply of oxygen and glucose, thereby maintaining metabolic homeostasis.

Functionally, the blood–brain barrier serves several critical roles. It protects by preventing the entry of toxins, pathogens, and many circulating immune cells. It maintains homeostasis by regulating ionic composition and neurotransmitter levels within the extracellular fluid of the brain. It enables selective transport of essential nutrients, including glucose, amino acids, and vitamins, while facilitating the removal of metabolic waste products through efflux transporters and the glymphatic system. In addition, it contributes to immune regulation by limiting the access of peripheral immune cells to the central nervous system, thereby preserving the unique immunological environment of the brain.

Despite its effectiveness, the blood–brain barrier is not uniformly present throughout the brain. Certain specialized regions, known as circumventricular organs, lack a typical barrier and instead possess fenestrated capillaries. These regions allow the brain to monitor and respond directly to changes in the composition of the blood. The area postrema functions as a chemoreceptor trigger zone for vomiting, detecting circulating toxins. The median eminence plays a critical role in hypothalamic hormone release into the portal circulation. The neurohypophysis, or posterior pituitary, allows direct secretion of hormones such as oxytocin and vasopressin into the bloodstream. The pineal gland, which secretes melatonin, also lies outside the strict confines of the blood–brain barrier.

Disruption or dysfunction of the blood–brain barrier has significant clinical implications. In infections such as meningitis, increased permeability of the barrier allows inflammatory cells and proteins to enter the cerebrospinal fluid, contributing to edema and neuronal injury. In encephalitis, infiltration of immune cells into the brain parenchyma reflects breakdown of barrier integrity. In stroke, ischemia leads to compromise of the barrier, resulting in vasogenic edema, while hemorrhagic stroke causes direct structural disruption. In neurodegenerative disorders such as Alzheimer's disease, impairment of barrier function may reduce clearance of toxic proteins such as amyloid beta, contributing to disease progression. In Parkinson's disease, alterations in barrier transport and associated neuroinflammation may play a role in neuronal degeneration.

The blood–brain barrier also presents a major challenge in pharmacotherapy. Many drugs, particularly large or hydrophilic molecules, are unable to cross the barrier in sufficient concentrations to exert therapeutic effects. Lipid-soluble substances diffuse more readily, but even these may be actively removed by efflux pumps. To overcome these limitations, various strategies have been developed, including direct intrathecal administration, the use of nanoparticle carriers, and receptor-mediated transport systems that exploit endogenous transport mechanisms.

In summary, the blood–brain barrier is a critical component of the central nervous system that preserves neural homeostasis through highly selective permeability and tight regulation of the brain's internal environment. Its structural complexity, functional precision, and integration within the neurovascular unit make it indispensable for normal brain function, while its disruption plays a central role in a wide range of neurological diseases.

Review Questions

Q1. Which glucose transporter mediates BBB glucose uptake?
Answer: GLUT1.

Q2. Name one circumventricular organ lacking a BBB.
Answer: Area postrema.

Q3. What type of edema results from BBB disruption in stroke?
Answer: Vasogenic edema.

Q4. Which cell type provides structural and trophic support to BBB endothelial cells?
Answer: Astrocytic endfeet.

Q5. Why is drug delivery to the CNS challenging?
Answer: Tight junctions and efflux pumps restrict the entry of most molecules.

Clinical Vignettes

Vignette 1 — Stroke and BBB Breakdown
A patient with MCA infarct develops cerebral edema.
Mechanism: BBB disruption → vasogenic edema.

Vignette 2 — Meningitis
A child with bacterial meningitis shows increased CSF protein.
Mechanism: BBB permeability increased, allowing plasma proteins to enter CSF.

Vignette 3 — Alzheimer's Disease
An elderly patient with progressive memory loss shows amyloid plaques.
Mechanism: BBB dysfunction impairs amyloidβ clearance.

Vignette 4 — Chemotherapy Challenge
A patient with brain metastasis fails systemic chemotherapy.
Mechanism: BBB prevents drug penetration.

References

1. Kandel ER, Schwartz JH, Jessell TM, Siegelbaum SA, Hudspeth AJ. *Principles of Neural Science*. 5th ed. McGraw-Hill; 2013.
2. Abbott NJ, Rönnbäck L, Hansson E. *Astrocyte–endothelial interactions at the blood–brain barrier*. Nat Rev Neurosci. 2006;7(1):4153.
3. Zlokovic BV. *The blood–brain barrier in health and chronic neurodegenerative disorders*. Neuron. 2008;57(2):178201.
4. Purves D, Augustine GJ, Fitzpatrick D, et al. *Neuroscience*. 6th ed. Oxford University Press; 2018.

Chapter 19

Somatosensory Pathways

Click here to view
Chapter Video: https://youtu.be/P6qocUCrmV8

Overview of the Somatosensory System

The somatosensory system is a highly organized and functionally sophisticated network responsible for conveying sensory information from the skin, muscles, tendons, joints, and deep tissues to the central nervous system. Through this system, the body perceives touch, pressure, vibration, pain, temperature, and proprioception. Despite the diversity of these sensory modalities, the system follows a remarkably consistent organizational plan throughout the neuraxis, reflecting a common structural and functional framework.

All major somatosensory pathways are built upon a fundamental three-neuron chain that extends from the peripheral receptor to the primary somatosensory cortex. The first-order neuron carries information from the receptor to the central nervous system, the second-order neuron decussates and ascends toward the thalamus, and the third-order neuron relays the signal from the thalamus to the cortex. This arrangement ensures that sensory information from one side of the body is ultimately represented in the contralateral cerebral hemisphere. Within the thalamus, relay occurs primarily through the ventral posterior nuclei, with the ventral posterolateral nucleus transmitting sensory input from the body and the ventral posteromedial nucleus conveying information from the face.

Primary sensory neurons are located in the dorsal root ganglia and are characteristically pseudo-unipolar. Each neuron possesses a peripheral process that detects stimuli through specialized receptors or free nerve endings, and a central process that enters the spinal cord via the dorsal root. This unique morphology allows rapid conduction of impulses without synaptic interruption at the level of the ganglion.

Somatosensory receptors are specialized according to the modality of stimulus they detect. Nociceptors and thermoreceptors consist of free nerve endings that respond to pain and temperature, respectively. Mechanoreceptors, in contrast, are structurally specialized to detect mechanical deformation. Meissner corpuscles, located in glabrous skin, mediate fine touch and two-point discrimination. Merkel cells, found in the epidermis, are sensitive to pressure and texture. Ruffini endings, located in the dermis, respond to skin stretch, while Pacinian corpuscles, situated in deeper tissues, detect vibration and deep pressure. Proprioceptive information arises from muscle spindles, which monitor muscle length, and Golgi tendon organs, which detect muscle tension. These mechanoreceptive and proprioceptive signals are typically transmitted by large, myelinated A beta fibers, which conduct impulses rapidly.

Sensory fibers are classified according to diameter, degree of myelination, and conduction velocity. In the alphabetic system, A fibers are myelinated and subdivided into A alpha fibers for proprioception, A beta fibers for touch and vibration, and A delta fibers for fast pain and temperature. B fibers are lightly myelinated and associated with autonomic function, whereas C fibers are unmyelinated and transmit slow pain and temperature. The alphanumeric system parallels this classification, designating Group I fibers as the largest and fastest, associated with muscle spindles, and Group IV fibers as the smallest and slowest, corresponding to unmyelinated pain fibers. In both systems, fiber size correlates directly with conduction velocity and functional modality.

Two principal ascending pathways convey somatic sensory information: the posterior column–medial lemniscus pathway and the anterolateral system. The posterior column–medial lemniscus pathway transmits modalities that require high spatial and temporal resolution, including fine touch, vibration, pressure, and conscious proprioception. **First-order neurons** enter the spinal cord and ascend ipsilaterally within the dorsal columns, which are organized somatotopically. The gracile fasciculus, located medially, carries information from the lower limb and lower trunk, whereas the cuneate fasciculus, positioned laterally, conveys input from the upper limb and upper trunk.

Second-order neurons reside in the nucleus gracilis and nucleus cuneatus of the caudal medulla. Their axons decussate as internal arcuate fibers and ascend as the medial lemniscus. As the pathway ascends through the brainstem, the orientation of the medial lemniscus changes, reflecting the reorganization of somatotopic representation. **Third-order neurons** are located in the ventral posterolateral nucleus of the thalamus and project to the primary somatosensory cortex, specifically Brodmann areas 3, 1, and 2 of the postcentral gyrus. This pathway is essential for discriminative sensation and plays a critical role in fine motor control and spatial awareness.

Somatosensory information from the face follows an analogous pathway through the trigeminal system. First-order neurons reside in the trigeminal ganglion, and their central processes enter the brainstem at the level of the pons. Second-order neurons in the principal sensory nucleus of the trigeminal nerve decussate and ascend as the trigeminal lemniscus alongside the medial lemniscus. These fibers terminate in the ventral posteromedial nucleus of the thalamus, which projects to the corresponding region of the primary somatosensory cortex. Together, the ventral posterolateral and ventral posteromedial nuclei serve as the principal thalamic relays for somatosensory information from the body and face, respectively.

The posterior column–medial lemniscus system mediates highly refined sensory functions, including two-point discrimination, stereognosis, graphesthesia, vibration sense, pressure perception, and conscious proprioception. Lesions affecting this pathway result in characteristic deficits such as sensory ataxia, hyporeflexia, astereognosis, and agraphesthesia. Loss of proprioceptive input also produces a positive Romberg sign, reflecting impaired postural stability.

In contrast, **the anterolateral system** conveys modalities that are protective and rapidly adaptive, including pain, temperature, and crude touch. These sensations are detected by free nerve endings and transmitted by A delta fibers, which carry fast, sharp, well-localized pain, and C fibers, which convey slow, dull, and poorly localized pain. The central processes of these fibers enter the spinal cord and immediately branch within Lissauer's tract, giving rise to ascending and descending collaterals.

Within the dorsal horn, A delta fibers primarily synapse in laminae I and V, contributing to the transmission of fast pain signals. C fibers synapse in lamina II, also known as the substantia gelatinosa, a key site for modulation of nociceptive input. Additional processing occurs in laminae III and IV, which receive non-noxious input, and in lamina V, where convergent input from multiple modalities contributes to phenomena such as referred pain. Deep dorsal horn neurons encode pain intensity and give rise to second-order neurons of the anterolateral system.

Second-order neurons decussate in the anterior white commissure within one to two spinal segments of their entry and ascend contralaterally in the anterolateral funiculus. Although traditionally divided into lateral and ventral spinothalamic tracts, these pathways collectively transmit all modalities of the anterolateral system.

The anterolateral system includes both direct and indirect pain pathways. The neospinothalamic pathway, mediated primarily by A delta fibers, transmits fast, well-localized pain to the ventral posterior nuclei of the thalamus and subsequently to the primary somatosensory cortex, enabling precise localization and discrimination. In contrast, the paleospinothalamic pathway is polysynaptic and mediated predominantly by C fibers. It projects to the reticular formation, medial thalamic nuclei, cingulate cortex, and other limbic structures, mediating the emotional, motivational, and autonomic components of pain.

In addition to these principal pathways, the anterolateral system gives rise to several collateral projections that contribute to the broader physiological and behavioral response to painful stimuli. Spinoreticular fibers influence arousal and autonomic responses, spinohypothalamic pathways link pain to neuroendocrine and autonomic regulation, and spinotectal fibers mediate orienting reflexes toward noxious stimuli.

In summary, the somatosensory system is an intricately organized network that integrates multiple modalities of sensation through distinct but complementary pathways. The posterior column–medial lemniscus system provides precise, discriminative sensory information, whereas the anterolateral system conveys protective and affective aspects of sensation. Together, these pathways enable the nervous system to interpret, localize, and respond appropriately to a wide range of external and internal stimuli.

Review Questions

Q1. A patient presents with dull, aching pain accompanied by emotional distress. Which pathway is responsible?
Answer: Paleospinothalamic pathway (C fibers → reticular formation → medial thalamus).

Q2. Pain and temperature from the face synapse first in which structure?
Answer: Spinal nucleus of the trigeminal nerve.

Q3. The dorsal spinocerebellar tract carries information from which nucleus?
Answer: Clarke's nucleus (C8–L3).

Q4. Which tract crosses twice before reaching the cerebellum?
Answer: Anterior spinocerebellar tract.

Q5. The trigeminal lemniscus terminates in which thalamic nucleus?
Answer: Ventral posterior medial (VPM) nucleus.

Q6. Which fibers form Lissauer's tract?
Answer: Adelta and C fibers.

Q7. A lesion of the anterior white commissure impairs which modalities?
Answer: Pain and temperature.

Q8. Upper limb unconscious proprioception synapses in which nucleus?
Answer: Lateral cuneate nucleus.

Q9. Which pathway mediates emotional and arousal components of pain?
Answer: Spinoreticular and spinothalamic projections to intralaminar and mediodorsal nuclei.

Q10. Loss of vibration sense, positive Romberg sign, and sensory ataxia indicate damage to which pathway?
Answer: Dorsal column–medial lemniscus system.

References

1. Snell's Clinical Neuroanatomy
Snell RS. *Clinical Neuroanatomy*. 8th ed. Wolters Kluwer.

2. Gray's Anatomy for Students
Drake RL, Vogl W, Mitchell AWM. *Gray's Anatomy for Students*. 4th ed. Elsevier.

3. Principles of Neural Science
Kandel ER, et al. *Principles of Neural Science*. 6th ed. McGraw-Hill.

Chapter 20
Motor System Organization

Click here to view
Chapter Video: https://youtu.be/tx2PlTr5ccE

Introduction to the Motor System

Voluntary movement represents one of the most refined and complex functions of the nervous system, requiring the coordinated integration of intention, planning, sensory feedback, and precise execution. Movements originate in the motor cortex, where they are consciously initiated, and are subsequently shaped and refined through experience and practice. With repetition, these movements become increasingly efficient and may evolve into highly skilled motor patterns. In contrast, reflex movements are rapid, involuntary responses to specific sensory stimuli. Their circuitry is largely hard-wired within the spinal cord and brainstem, allowing for immediate protective or postural responses without conscious involvement. Classic examples include the stretch reflex, initiated by activation of muscle spindles, and the withdrawal reflex, triggered by nociceptive input from the skin.

Effective motor control depends on the integration of several essential components. Volition provides the conscious drive to initiate movement, while coordination ensures that the appropriate muscles are activated in the correct sequence and intensity. Proprioception supplies continuous feedback regarding the position and movement of body parts, enabling real-time adjustments. Postural mechanisms maintain balance and stability, and unconscious processing within the cerebellum and spinal cord refines movements automatically. Sensory input from muscle receptors, including information about muscle length, rate of stretch, and tension, is indispensable for the continuous modulation of motor output.

The motor system is organized hierarchically into multiple functional levels. At the highest level, the motor cortex initiates voluntary movement and encodes parameters such as force, direction, and speed. Adjacent motor association areas are responsible for planning complex sequences and integrating sensory information with motor intention. Brainstem centers, including the vestibular nuclei, reticular formation, red nucleus, and tectum, regulate posture, balance, and basic movement patterns. The spinal cord serves as the final execution level, where alpha motor neurons directly innervate skeletal muscle and mediate reflex activity. In addition to this vertical hierarchy, two critical side-loop systems modulate motor function. The basal ganglia maintain purposeful movement and suppress unwanted activity, whereas the cerebellum coordinates timing, precision, and force while maintaining equilibrium. Both systems communicate with the cerebral cortex through the thalamus, forming feedback circuits essential for smooth and coordinated movement.

Nerve fibers involved in motor and sensory transmission are classified according to their diameter, degree of myelination, and conduction velocity. In the alphabetic system, A fibers are myelinated and subdivided into A alpha fibers, which innervate extrafusal muscle fibers and convey proprioceptive information; A beta fibers, which transmit touch and pressure; A gamma fibers, which supply intrafusal fibers of the muscle spindle; and A delta fibers, which carry fast pain and temperature. B fibers are lightly myelinated autonomic fibers, whereas C fibers are unmyelinated and conduct slow pain and temperature. The alphanumeric system parallels this classification, with Type I fibers corresponding to large, rapidly conducting proprioceptive afferents, Type II fibers mediating touch and pressure, and Types III and IV corresponding to fast and slow pain fibers, respectively. These systems highlight the close relationship between fiber size, conduction velocity, and functional modality.

A key sensory organ in motor control is the muscle spindle, a specialized proprioceptor embedded within skeletal muscle. It consists of intrafusal muscle fibers surrounded by the larger extrafusal fibers that constitute the bulk of the muscle. The spindle is innervated by gamma motor neurons, which regulate its sensitivity, while extrafusal fibers are supplied by alpha motor neurons responsible for contraction. Sensory innervation is provided by Ia and II afferent fibers. The muscle spindle detects both muscle length and the rate of change of length, providing critical information for the regulation of muscle tone, posture, and reflex activity. Primary endings respond dynamically to stretch, whereas secondary endings provide information about static muscle length.

Closely related to the muscle spindle is the Golgi tendon organ, which monitors muscle tension. Together, these receptors form the basis of reflex mechanisms that protect muscles and ensure smooth control of force. The stretch reflex, or myotatic reflex, is a monosynaptic pathway in which Ia afferents synapse directly on alpha motor neurons, producing contraction of the stretched muscle and preventing overstretching. In contrast, the inverse stretch reflex mediated by Golgi tendon organs is polysynaptic; Ib afferents activate inhibitory interneurons that suppress alpha motor neuron activity, resulting in muscle relaxation and protection against excessive tension. These opposing mechanisms operate in a coordinated manner, producing reciprocal interactions between agonist and antagonist muscles that stabilize movement and prevent injury.

The stretch reflex arc exemplifies the simplicity and efficiency of spinal reflex circuits. Sensory input from the muscle spindle is transmitted via Ia afferents to the spinal cord, where it directly excites alpha motor neurons supplying the same muscle. Simultaneously, inhibitory interneurons suppress activity in antagonist muscles, a process known as reciprocal inhibition. Gamma motor neurons adjust spindle sensitivity, ensuring that the system remains responsive during changes in muscle length. This reflex is fundamental for maintaining posture and enabling smooth, coordinated movement.

Protective reflexes are exemplified by the withdrawal reflex, a polysynaptic response triggered by painful cutaneous stimuli. Activation of nociceptors leads to excitation of flexor muscles and inhibition of extensors on the affected side, resulting in rapid withdrawal of the limb. To maintain balance, a complementary crossed extensor reflex activates extensors and inhibits flexors in the contralateral limb, providing postural support during withdrawal.

At the cellular level, all motor commands ultimately converge at the neuromuscular junction, the specialized synapse between motor neurons and skeletal muscle fibers. Each alpha motor neuron innervates multiple muscle fibers, forming a motor unit. Small motor units allow fine, precise control, whereas large motor units generate powerful, gross movements. The neuromuscular junction is structurally adapted for rapid and reliable transmission. The presynaptic terminal contains voltage-gated calcium channels and synaptic vesicles filled with acetylcholine. The synaptic cleft contains acetylcholinesterase, which rapidly degrades the neurotransmitter, while the postsynaptic membrane, or motor end plate, is highly folded and densely packed with nicotinic acetylcholine receptors.

Neuromuscular transmission begins with the arrival of an action potential at the presynaptic terminal, leading to calcium influx and vesicle fusion. Acetylcholine is released into the synaptic cleft, diffuses across to the postsynaptic membrane, and binds to nicotinic receptors, opening cation channels and generating an end plate potential. If this potential reaches threshold, it triggers a muscle action potential, resulting in contraction. Rapid breakdown of acetylcholine ensures precise control and prevents continuous stimulation.

The physiology of the neuromuscular junction underlies the action of several pharmacological agents. Non-depolarizing neuromuscular blockers act as competitive antagonists at nicotinic receptors, preventing acetylcholine binding and producing flaccid paralysis. Depolarizing agents, in contrast, mimic acetylcholine but resist degradation, leading to prolonged depolarization and eventual paralysis following initial muscle fasciculations. These agents are widely used in anesthesia and critical care.

Disorders of neuromuscular transmission illustrate the importance of this system. Myasthenia gravis is an autoimmune condition characterized by antibodies against postsynaptic acetylcholine receptors, resulting in reduced end-plate potentials and fatigable muscle weakness. In Lambert–Eaton myasthenic syndrome, antibodies target presynaptic calcium channels, impairing acetylcholine release and causing proximal weakness that improves with repeated activity. Botulism, caused by a neurotoxin that blocks vesicle fusion, leads to profound paralysis by preventing acetylcholine release.

Alterations in muscle tone provide important clinical clues to the site of neurological lesions. Lower motor neuron lesions result in flaccidity, characterized by decreased tone, muscle atrophy, and loss of reflexes. In contrast, upper motor neuron lesions produce spasticity, marked by increased tone, hyperreflexia, and velocity-dependent resistance to movement due to loss of inhibitory control over spinal reflexes. Basal ganglia disorders lead to rigidity, which is independent of movement velocity and often exhibits a "lead pipe" or "cogwheel" quality. Cerebellar lesions typically produce hypotonia and incoordination.

A classic manifestation of upper motor neuron dysfunction is the clasp knife phenomenon, in which initial resistance to passive movement is followed by a sudden release, resembling the closing of a pocketknife. This reflects the interplay between exaggerated stretch reflex activity and inhibitory influences mediated by Golgi tendon organs.

In summary, the motor system is a complex and hierarchically organized network that integrates cortical intention, subcortical modulation, spinal execution, and peripheral feedback. Through the coordinated activity of reflex circuits, proprioceptive mechanisms, and neuromuscular transmission, it enables the precise control of movement, posture, and muscle tone essential for normal function.

Review Questions

Q1. A patient with proximal muscle weakness improves after repeated contractions. Which disorder is most likely?
Answer: Lambert–Eaton myasthenic syndrome.

Q2. Botulinum toxin causes paralysis by blocking which process?
Answer: Presynaptic acetylcholine release.

Q3. Increased resistance to passive movement that varies with speed is characteristic of which condition?
Answer: Spasticity (UMN lesion).

Q4. Rigidity constant throughout the range of motion suggests dysfunction of which structure?
Answer: Basal ganglia.

Q5. Loss of reflexes, decreased tone, and muscle atrophy indicate which type of lesion?
Answer: Lower motor neuron lesion.

Q6. The claspknife phenomenon is associated with which deficit?
Answer: Spasticity due to UMN damage.

Q7. In Lambert–Eaton syndrome, antibodies target which channel?
Answer: Presynaptic voltage-gated calcium channels.

Q8. Opening of presynaptic Ca^{2+} channels at the NMJ directly triggers which event?
Answer: Fusion of ACh-containing vesicles with the presynaptic membrane.

Q9. A competitive antagonist of nicotinic ACh receptors produces which effect?
Answer: Flaccid paralysis without depolarization.

Q10. Which enzyme terminates ACh action in the synaptic cleft?
Answer: Acetylcholinesterase.

Q11. Fatigable weakness improving with AChE inhibitors indicates what pathology?
Answer: Myasthenia gravis.

Q12. Depolarizing neuromuscular blockers produce paralysis by which mechanism?
Answer: Sustained depolarization of the motor end plate.

Q13. The end plate potential is generated by activation of which receptor?
Answer: Nicotinic ligand-gated ion channels.

Q14. Which neurotransmitter is released at the NMJ?
Answer: Acetylcholine.

Q15. Which receptor detects the **rate** of muscle stretch?
Answer: Ia fibers of the muscle spindle (annulospiral endings).

16. Spasticity with a claspknife response indicates a lesion in which pathway?
Answer: Corticospinal tract (UMN).

Q17. Flaccid paralysis, fasciculations, and areflexia localize the lesion where?
Answer: Lower motor neuron.

References:

1. Snell's Clinical Neuroanatomy
   Snell RS. *Clinical Neuroanatomy*. 8th ed. Wolters Kluwer.
2. Gray's Anatomy for Students
   Drake RL, Vogl W, Mitchell AWM. *Gray's Anatomy for Students*. 4th ed. Elsevier.
3. Principles of Neural Science
   Kandel ER, et al. *Principles of Neural Science*. 6th ed. McGraw-Hill.

Chapter 21

Descending Motor Pathways Pyramidal and Extrapyramidal Systems, and Clinical Correlates

Click here to view
Chapter Video: https://youtu.be/RqDe-SPVRHA

Introduction

Voluntary movement is executed through two principal descending motor systems: the pyramidal and extrapyramidal systems. These systems function in a complementary and integrated manner to produce coordinated, purposeful movement. The pyramidal system, comprising the corticospinal and corticobulbar tracts, is primarily responsible for precise, skilled, and fractionated voluntary movements, especially those involving distal musculature such as the fingers. In contrast, the extrapyramidal system consists of descending pathways originating from brainstem motor nuclei and plays a crucial role in maintaining posture, balance, muscle tone, and automatic adjustments that accompany voluntary actions. Together, these systems ensure that movement is not only accurate but also stable and adaptable to changing environmental demands.

The pyramidal system originates predominantly from the primary motor cortex, specifically Brodmann area 4, where large pyramidal neurons known as Betz cells reside in layer V. Additional contributions arise from the premotor cortex, supplementary motor area, and somatosensory cortex, reflecting the integration of planning and sensory feedback into motor execution. The corticospinal tract descends from these cortical areas through the corona radiata and converges within the posterior limb of the internal capsule, occupying its anterior two-thirds. It then continues through the cerebral peduncles in the midbrain, traverses the basis pontis, and forms the medullary pyramids in the ventral medulla.

At the caudal medulla, approximately 90 percent of corticospinal fibers decussate in the pyramidal decussation to form the lateral corticospinal tract, which descends in the lateral column of the spinal cord. The remaining fibers continue as the anterior corticospinal tract and cross segmentally near their level of termination. These fibers ultimately synapse either directly on alpha and gamma motor neurons or via interneurons in the ventral horn. Functionally, the corticospinal tract enables precise voluntary movements, particularly those requiring fine motor control and independent finger movements, and also modulates spinal reflex activity.

The corticobulbar tract, the second major component of the pyramidal system, carries motor commands from the cortex to the motor nuclei of cranial nerves in the brainstem. These include nuclei associated with ocular movements, mastication, facial expression, swallowing, phonation, and tongue movement. Most cranial nerve motor nuclei receive bilateral cortical innervation, which provides a degree of redundancy and functional preservation. However, notable exceptions include the lower facial muscles supplied by the facial nerve and the genioglossus muscle supplied by the hypoglossal nerve, both of which receive predominantly contralateral cortical input. This pattern explains important clinical distinctions: upper motor neuron lesions affecting the facial nerve result in weakness of the contralateral lower face with sparing of the forehead, whereas lower motor neuron lesions produce complete ipsilateral facial paralysis. Similarly, upper motor neuron lesions of the hypoglossal pathway cause the tongue to deviate away from the lesion, while lower motor neuron lesions result in deviation toward the side of the lesion, often accompanied by fasciculations.

In contrast to the pyramidal system, the extrapyramidal system consists of several descending tracts that originate from brainstem nuclei and are heavily influenced by inputs from the cerebellum, cerebral cortex, and sensory systems, including visual, vestibular, and proprioceptive pathways. These tracts primarily control axial and proximal musculature, thereby maintaining posture and facilitating coordinated movement.

The rubrospinal tract arises from the red nucleus in the midbrain and decussates almost immediately after its origin. It descends adjacent to the corticospinal tract and facilitates flexor muscle activity while inhibiting extensor muscles. Although less prominent in humans than in other species, it contributes to distal limb coordination. The tectospinal tract originates from the superior colliculus and mediates reflexive movements of the head and neck in response to visual stimuli, thereby coordinating eye and head orientation.

The vestibulospinal tracts originate from the medial and lateral vestibular nuclei and play a central role in maintaining balance and posture. The medial vestibulospinal tract primarily stabilizes the head and neck, while the lateral vestibulospinal tract facilitates extensor muscle tone to support upright posture. The reticulospinal tracts, arising from the pontine and medullary reticular formation, modulate muscle tone, coordinate posture and locomotion, and integrate signals from the corticospinal system and cerebellum. These pathways are essential for the automatic adjustments that accompany voluntary movement.

Lesions affecting descending motor pathways produce characteristic clinical patterns depending on whether the damage involves upper motor neurons or lower motor neurons. Upper motor neuron lesions occur in structures such as the motor cortex, corona radiata, internal capsule, brainstem above the level of cranial nerve nuclei, and the spinal cord above the anterior horn cells. These lesions result in spastic weakness, increased muscle tone, hyperreflexia, clonus, and the presence of a Babinski sign. Muscle atrophy is typically minimal and reflects disuse rather than denervation. A hallmark of upper motor neuron dysfunction is the loss of fine motor control. For example, lesions in the internal capsule often produce dense contralateral hemiplegia due to the compact arrangement of descending fibers, whereas cortical lesions may produce more selective deficits accompanied by higher cortical signs such as aphasia or neglect. Brainstem lesions characteristically produce "crossed findings," in which ipsilateral cranial nerve deficits are associated with contralateral limb weakness.

Lower motor neuron lesions, in contrast, involve the final common pathway, including anterior horn cells, cranial nerve motor nuclei, peripheral nerves, neuromuscular junctions, and muscle fibers. These lesions produce flaccid weakness, decreased muscle tone, hyporeflexia or areflexia, fasciculations, and marked muscle atrophy due to denervation. Unlike upper motor neuron lesions, there is no Babinski sign. In the context of stroke, lower motor neuron signs are typically observed when cranial nerve motor nuclei are directly affected by brainstem infarction.

The distinction between upper and lower motor neuron lesions is fundamental to clinical localization. Upper motor neuron lesions tend to affect groups of muscles and produce spastic paralysis, whereas lower motor neuron lesions affect individual muscles or muscle groups and produce flaccid paralysis with significant atrophy. These contrasting patterns provide critical diagnostic clues during neurological examination.

Voluntary movement ultimately reflects the integration of multiple neural systems. The pyramidal system provides the capacity for precise, fractionated movement, while the extrapyramidal system ensures appropriate posture, tone, and automatic adjustments. The cerebellum contributes timing, coordination, and error correction, whereas the basal ganglia are involved in the initiation, scaling, and selection of movement. All of these systems converge on alpha and gamma motor neurons, which serve as the final common pathway for motor output. Through this complex and highly coordinated network, the nervous system produces smooth, purposeful, and adaptive movements essential for interaction with the environment.

Review Questions

Q1. Where do corticospinal fibers decussate?
Answer: Caudal medulla (pyramidal decussation).

Q2. Which cranial nerve nuclei receive only contralateral corticobulbar input?
Answer: Lower CN VII nucleus and CN XII nucleus.

Q3. What is the hallmark of a UMN lesion?
Spasticity with hyperreflexia and Babinski sign.

Q4. Which tract facilitates flexor muscles?
Answer: Rubrospinal tract.

Q5. Which descending pathway mediates reflexive head turning toward visual stimuli?
Answer: Tectospinal tract.

Q6. What is the primary function of the lateral corticospinal tract?
Answer: Skilled voluntary movement of distal limbs.

Q7. What distinguishes UMN from LMN facial weakness?
Answer: UMN → lower face only; LMN → entire ipsilateral face.

Clinical Vignettes

Vignette 1 — Internal Capsule Stroke
A 72-year-old man develops sudden right-sided weakness of the face, arm, and leg with increased tone, brisk reflexes, and Babinski sign.
Diagnosis: Left UMN lesion (internal capsule infarct).

Vignette 2 — Bell's Palsy
Complete paralysis of the left side of the face, including the forehead.
Diagnosis: LMN lesion of CN VII.

Vignette 3 — Hypoglossal Lesion
Tongue deviates to the left after a left medullary infarct.
Diagnosis: Left LMN lesion of CN XII.

Vignette 4 — Rubrospinal Dysfunction
Midbrain stroke with impaired distal limb coordination and slowed movement.
Diagnosis: Red nucleus involvement.

Vignette 5 — Tectospinal Reflex
A sudden loud noise triggers reflexive head and eye turning toward the source.
Explanation: Activation of the tectospinal pathway

References

1. Snell's Clinical Neuroanatomy
   Snell RS. *Clinical Neuroanatomy*. 8th ed. Wolters Kluwer.
2. Gray's Anatomy for Students
   Drake RL, Vogl W, Mitchell AWM. *Gray's Anatomy for Students*. 4th ed. Elsevier.
3. Neuroanatomy Through Clinical Cases
   Blumenfeld H. *Neuroanatomy Through Clinical Cases*. 3rd ed. Sinauer Associates.
4. Principles of Neural Science
   Kandel ER, et al. *Principles of Neural Science*. 6th ed. McGraw-Hill.

Chapter 22

Cerebellum and Vascular Syndromes (Anatomy, Functional Organization, and Cellular Architecture)

Click here to view
Chapter Video: https://youtu.be/WuE6rBJ_KeM

The cerebellum, a major component of the hindbrain, plays a central role in the coordination, precision, and timing of movement. Although it does not initiate voluntary activity, it continuously refines motor output, ensuring that movements are smooth, accurate, and appropriately scaled. In addition to its essential contributions to posture, gait, and eye movements, the cerebellum also participates in higher-order cognitive and affective processes through its extensive connections with the cerebral cortex. Despite these broader roles, its motor functions remain the most clinically significant and best understood.

Anatomically, the cerebellum is situated within the posterior cranial fossa, separated from the occipital lobes by the tentorium cerebelli. It lies posterior to the pons and medulla, from which it is separated by the fourth ventricle. Its surface is highly convoluted, consisting of numerous narrow, transverse folds known as folia, which greatly increase the cortical surface area and contribute to its characteristic laminated appearance.

Structurally, the cerebellum is organized in a manner analogous to the cerebrum. A peripheral layer of Gray matter forms the cerebellar cortex, beneath which lies a core of white matter containing afferent and efferent fibers. Embedded within this white matter are the deep cerebellar nuclei, which serve as the principal output stations of the cerebellum. These three components—the cortex, white matter tracts, and deep nuclei—operate in concert to integrate sensory inputs, modulate motor commands, and maintain equilibrium.

Communication between the cerebellum and the brainstem occurs through three paired cerebellar peduncles, each with distinct functional roles. The superior cerebellar peduncle serves primarily as an efferent pathway, conveying cerebellar output to the midbrain, particularly to the red nucleus and the ventrolateral nucleus of the thalamus. The middle cerebellar peduncle is exclusively afferent and represents the largest input pathway, transmitting pontocerebellar fibers from the contralateral pontine nuclei, which themselves receive input from the cerebral cortex. The inferior cerebellar peduncle contains both afferent and efferent fibers and connects the cerebellum to the medulla, carrying proprioceptive information from the spinal cord as well as input from vestibular nuclei.

The cerebellum is divided into two hemispheres connected by a midline structure known as the vermis. Its surface is further subdivided by major fissures, including the primary fissure, which separates the anterior and posterior lobes, and the posterolateral fissure, which demarcates the flocculonodular lobe. The flocculonodular lobe, composed of the flocculus and nodule, is the smallest subdivision and is functionally associated with vestibular control and balance.

Functionally, the cerebellum is organized into three major divisions, each defined by its inputs, outputs, and physiological roles. The vestibulocerebellum, corresponding to the flocculonodular lobe, receives input from the vestibular apparatus and vestibular nuclei and projects back to these nuclei. It is primarily responsible for maintaining balance, equilibrium, and the coordination of eye movements, particularly through its influence on the vestibulo-ocular reflex. The spinocerebellum, comprising the vermis and intermediate (paravermal) zones, receives extensive proprioceptive input from the spinal cord as well as input from the trigeminal, visual, and auditory systems. It regulates posture, gait, and ongoing limb movements by influencing axial and proximal musculature. The Cerebrocerebellum, located in the lateral hemispheres, receives input from the cerebral cortex via pontine nuclei and projects to the dentate nucleus, which in turn communicates with the motor and premotor cortices through the thalamus. This division is essential for the planning, timing, and coordination of skilled voluntary movements.

Within the cerebellar white matter lie four pairs of deep cerebellar nuclei arranged from lateral to medial as the dentate, emboliform, globose, and fastigial nuclei. Each nucleus corresponds functionally to a specific cerebellar division. The dentate nucleus is associated with the Cerebrocerebellum and plays a major role in motor planning and coordination. The emboliform and globose nuclei, collectively referred to as the interposed nuclei, are linked to the spinocerebellum and regulate ongoing movements. The fastigial nucleus is connected to the vermis and vestibulocerebellum and is primarily involved in balance and axial control. These nuclei receive inhibitory input from Purkinje cells of the cerebellar cortex and send excitatory projections to motor centers in the brainstem and thalamus.

The cerebellar cortex itself exhibits a highly uniform three-layered structure. The outer molecular layer contains parallel fibers, which are the axons of granule cells, along with inhibitory interneurons such as stellate and basket cells. This layer is a major site of synaptic integration. Beneath it lies the Purkinje cell layer, a single row of large, flask-shaped neurons whose dendritic arbors extend into the molecular layer. Purkinje cells are the sole output neurons of the cerebellar cortex and exert inhibitory effects on the deep cerebellar nuclei through the neurotransmitter gamma-aminobutyric acid. These cells receive two distinct types of excitatory input: climbing fibers from the inferior olivary nucleus, which provide powerful, highly specific stimulation, and parallel fibers from granule cells, which provide more diffuse input. The innermost granule cell layer contains densely packed excitatory granule cells and inhibitory Golgi cells. Granule cell axons ascend to the molecular layer, where they bifurcate to form parallel fibers, thereby linking multiple Purkinje cells within a functional network.

Cerebellar afferent systems are broadly categorized into mossy fibers and climbing fibers, which together form the basis of cerebellar information processing. Mossy fibers arise from diverse sources, including the cerebral cortex via pontine nuclei, the spinal cord, vestibular structures, reticular formation, and trigeminal sensory nuclei. They synapse on granule cells in the granular layer, and through the parallel fiber system, indirectly influence Purkinje cells. These fibers provide a wide array of contextual sensory and motor information. In contrast, climbing fibers originate exclusively from the contralateral inferior olivary nucleus and form powerful, direct synaptic connections with Purkinje cells. Each climbing fiber wraps around the dendritic tree of a small number of Purkinje neurons, producing strong and precisely timed excitation.

Functionally, climbing fibers are critically involved in motor learning. They act as error signals, becoming active when there is a discrepancy between intended and actual movement. Their activation induces long-term depression at parallel fiber–Purkinje cell synapses, weakening those synaptic inputs that contributed to the error. This synaptic plasticity allows the cerebellum to update its internal models, thereby improving the accuracy and efficiency of future movements. Through this mechanism, the cerebellum serves as a computational comparator, continuously evaluating motor commands against sensory feedback.

Purkinje cells integrate inputs from mossy and climbing fibers and project inhibitory signals to the deep cerebellar nuclei. The pattern of these projections is highly organized: the vermis projects to the fastigial nucleus, the intermediate zone projects to the interposed nuclei, and the lateral hemispheres project to the dentate nucleus. The flocculonodular lobe projects both to the fastigial nucleus and directly to the vestibular nuclei. The deep nuclei then transmit excitatory output to motor centers in the brainstem and thalamus, thereby influencing descending motor pathways and cortical motor areas.

The cerebellum plays a crucial role in integrating proprioceptive and vestibular information. Proprioceptive input from muscle spindles, Golgi tendon organs, and joint receptors provides continuous information about limb position and movement, while vestibular input from the semicircular canals and otolith organs conveys information about head position and motion in space. By integrating these inputs, the cerebellum maintains posture, coordinates voluntary movement, and adjusts motor output in real time. Its communication with the motor cortex via the dentato-rubro-thalamic pathway further ensures that planned movements are executed with precision and adaptability.

Recent advances have expanded the understanding of cerebellar function beyond motor coordination. The recognition of cerebellar cognitive affective syndrome has highlighted the cerebellum's role in executive function, language, visuospatial processing, and emotional regulation, particularly in lesions involving the posterior lobe. Functional imaging studies have reinforced its role in prediction and error correction, emphasizing its function as a dynamic computational system. Additionally, the vulnerability of Purkinje cells to hypoxic and metabolic injury has provided insight into patterns of cerebellar damage observed in neonatal and metabolic disorders. Modern imaging techniques also allow more precise characterization of cerebellar atrophy, aiding in the diagnosis of hereditary ataxias.

In summary, the cerebellum is an essential integrative structure that refines motor activity through complex afferent and efferent circuits. By continuously comparing intended movement with actual performance and adjusting output accordingly, it ensures that motor behavior is smooth, coordinated, and adaptive to changing demands.

Review Questions

Q1. Which cerebellar peduncle carries the major efferent output?
Answer: Superior cerebellar peduncle.

Q2. What neurotransmitter is used by Purkinje cells?
Answer: GABA.

Q3. Which deep nucleus corresponds to the Cerebrocerebellum?
Answer: Dentate nucleus.

Q4. What is the primary function of the flocculonodular lobe?
Answer: Balance, equilibrium, and control of eye movements.

Q5. Which fibers mediate error correction during motor learning?
Answer: Climbing fibers from the inferior olivary nucleus.

Q6. What is the output pathway of the lateral cerebellar hemisphere?
Answer: Dentatorubrothalamic pathway.

Q7. Which cerebellar lesion produces truncal ataxia?
Answer: Flocculonodular lobe (vestibulocerebellum) lesion.

Clinical Vignettes

Vignette 1 Spinocerebellar Lesion

A patient presents with a wide-based gait, intention tremor, and dysmetria of the right arm. Proprioceptive pathways are intact.
Diagnosis: Right intermediate zone (spinocerebellum) lesion.

Vignette 2 Vestibulocerebellar Dysfunction

A 6-year-old child has difficulty maintaining balance, frequent falls, and horizontal nystagmus. MRI shows a lesion in the flocculonodular lobe.
Diagnosis: Vestibulocerebellar syndrome.

Vignette 3 Cerebrocerebellar Lesion

A pianist develops difficulty performing rapid alternating finger movements and shows delayed initiation of voluntary movement.
Diagnosis: Lateral hemisphere (Cerebrocerebellum) lesion.

Vignette 4 Purkinje Cell Vulnerability

A patient with severe hypoglycemia becomes comatose. MRI later shows selective cerebellar cortical injury.

Explanation: Purkinje cells are highly sensitive to metabolic stress.

Vignette 5 Inferior Olivary Dysfunction

A patient with a stroke involving the inferior olive shows impaired motor learning and an inability to adapt to prism-induced visual distortion.

Diagnosis: Loss of climbing fiber–mediated error correction.

References

1. Haines, D. E. *Neuroanatomy: An Atlas of Structures, Sections, and Systems.* Wolters Kluwer.
   Detailed coverage of cerebellar anatomy, peduncles, deep nuclei, and cortical layers.
2. Kandel, E. R., Schwartz, J. H., Jessell, T. M., et al. *Principles of Neural Science.* McGraw-Hill.
   Authoritative explanations of cerebellar circuitry, climbing/mossy fiber systems, and motor learning.
3. Voogd, J., & Glickstein, M. "The Anatomy of the Cerebellum." *Trends in Neurosciences.*
   Classic review of cerebellar organization, afferent–efferent pathways, and functional zones.
4. Schmahmann, J. D. *The Cerebellum and Cognition.* Academic Press.
   Foundational text describing the cerebellar cognitive affective syndrome (CCAS) and nonmotor functions.
5. Ito, M. "Control of Mental Activities by Internal Models in the Cerebellum." *Nature Reviews Neuroscience.*
   Seminal work on predictive modeling, error correction, and LTD mechanisms.

Chapter 23

The Visual Pathway: Anatomy, Functional Organization, and Clinical Correlates

Click here to view
Chapter Video: https://youtu.be/O3jw1_-icNc

Vision begins in the retina, where specialized photoreceptors—rods and cones—convert light energy into electrical signals. These signals are transmitted to retinal ganglion cells, whose axons converge to form the optic nerve, the first component of the visual pathway. From this point onward, visual information is conveyed through a precisely organized sequence of neural structures, including the optic chiasm, optic tract, lateral geniculate nucleus of the thalamus, optic radiations, and ultimately the primary visual cortex and associated Extrastriate regions. Through this pathway, raw light input is transformed into meaningful perception, encompassing shape, color, motion, depth, and spatial relationships.

An essential feature of the visual system is its orderly representation of the visual field. Light entering the eye is refracted by the cornea and lens to form an inverted image on the retina. The visual field is divided into right and left hemifields, each further subdivided into upper and lower quadrants. Importantly, each hemifield is processed by both eyes but through different halves of the retina. The left visual field is projected onto the right temporal retina and left nasal retina, while the right visual field is projected onto the left temporal retina and right nasal retina. The central region, where both eyes' visual fields overlap, constitutes the binocular field and is critical for depth perception.

The axons of retinal ganglion cells exit the eye at the optic disc to form the optic nerve, which passes through the optic canal into the cranial cavity. At the optic chiasm, a crucial partial decussation occurs: fibers from the nasal halves of the retina cross to the opposite side, while fibers from the temporal halves remain uncrossed. This arrangement ensures that each optic tract carries information from the contralateral visual field. Clinically, the optic chiasm is closely related to the pituitary gland, and compression by a pituitary adenoma classically produces bitemporal hemianopia due to selective involvement of crossing nasal fibers.

Beyond the chiasm, each optic tract conveys visual information to several subcortical targets, the most important of which is the lateral geniculate nucleus (LGN) of the thalamus. Additional projections reach the superior colliculus, which mediates reflexive eye and head movements; the pretectal nucleus, which is involved in the pupillary light reflex; and the suprachiasmatic nucleus, which regulates circadian rhythms.

The pupillary light reflex exemplifies a subcortical visual pathway. Light entering one eye is transmitted via the optic nerve and tract to the pretectal nucleus, which projects bilaterally to the Edinger–Westphal nuclei. From there, parasympathetic fibers travel with the oculomotor nerve to the ciliary ganglion and then to the constrictor pupillae muscles. As a result, illumination of one eye produces constriction of both pupils, a phenomenon known as the consensual light reflex.

The lateral geniculate nucleus serves as the principal relay station for visual information en route to the cortex. It is organized into six distinct layers, each receiving input from specific retinal sources. The magnocellular layers, which are the deeper layers, process motion and depth, whereas the parvocellular layers process fine detail, color, and form. This segregation allows parallel processing of different aspects of the visual scene.

From the LGN, axons project to the occipital lobe via the optic radiations. These fibers fan out around the lateral ventricles and are divided into two major pathways. The inferior fibers, known as Meyer's loop, sweep anteriorly into the temporal lobe before turning posteriorly to the occipital cortex; they carry information from the superior visual field. Lesions in this region produce a contralateral superior quadrantanopia, often described as a "pie in the sky" defect. In contrast, the superior fibers pass more directly through the parietal lobe and carry information from the inferior visual field; lesions here result in contralateral inferior quadrantanopia.

The primary visual cortex (V1), located along the banks of the calcarine sulcus in the occipital lobe, receives and processes visual input from the contralateral visual field. This cortex is organized retinotopically, meaning that adjacent regions of the retina are represented in adjacent regions of the cortex. A distinctive feature of V1 is the line of Gennari, a dense band of myelinated fibers visible within layer IV. At this level, basic visual attributes such as orientation, contrast, and spatial frequency are analyzed.

Beyond the primary visual cortex, visual processing becomes increasingly complex as information is distributed to the Extrastriate visual areas (V2–V5). These regions are organized into two major functional streams. **The dorsal stream**, often referred to as the "where pathway", projects to the posterior parietal cortex and is responsible for processing motion, spatial relationships, and visuomotor integration. Lesions in this pathway can result in hemispatial neglect, a condition in which the patient fails to attend to the contralateral side of space.

In contrast, **the ventral stream**, or the "what pathway", projects to the inferior temporal cortex and is involved in object recognition, color perception, and form analysis. Damage to this pathway leads to disorders such as visual agnosia, in which objects cannot be recognized visually despite intact vision, and prosopagnosia, the inability to recognize familiar faces, typically associated with lesions of the fusiform gyrus.

Thus, the visual pathway represents a highly organized and hierarchical system that transforms simple photic stimuli into rich perceptual experiences. Its precise anatomical arrangement not only enables efficient processing of visual information but also allows clinicians to localize lesions with remarkable accuracy based on characteristic visual field deficits and associated neurological signs.

Review Questions

Q1. Which retinal fibers decussate at the optic chiasm?
Answer: Nasal retinal fibers.

Q2. What visual deficit results from a pituitary adenoma compressing the chiasm?
Answer: Bitemporal hemianopia.

Q3. Which lobe contains Meyer's loop?
Answer: Temporal lobe.

Q4. What is the function of the dorsal visual stream?
Answer: Motion detection and spatial awareness.

Q5. What is the hallmark of a V1 lesion?
Answer: Contralateral homonymous hemianopia (often with macular sparing).

Q6. Which nucleus mediates the pupillary light reflex?
Answer: Pretectal nucleus → Edinger–Westphal nucleus.

Q7. Which LGN layers receive input from the temporal retina?
Answer: Layers 2, 3, and 5.

Clinical Vignettes

Vignette 1 Chiasmal Compression

A 45-year-old woman with a pituitary macroadenoma reports difficulty seeing objects in her peripheral vision. Visual field testing shows loss of temporal fields bilaterally.
Diagnosis: Bitemporal hemianopia.

Vignette 2 Temporal Lobe Lesion

A patient with a left temporal lobe tumor has difficulty seeing objects in the upper right quadrant of the visual field.
Diagnosis: Right superior quadrantanopia ("pie in the sky").

Vignette 3 Parietal Lesion

A stroke patient ignores objects on the left side of space and even neglects the left side of their own body.
Diagnosis: Right parietal lobe lesion → hemispatial neglect (dorsal stream).

Vignette 4 Ventral Stream Injury

A patient can describe an object by touch but cannot identify it visually.
Diagnosis: Visual agnosia (ventral stream lesion).

Vignette 5 Optic Tract Lesion

A patient with a right optic tract lesion presents with left homonymous hemianopia.
Explanation: The right optic tract carries left visual field information.

References

1. Snell's Clinical Neuroanatomy
   Snell RS. *Clinical Neuroanatomy*. 8th ed. Wolters Kluwer.
2. Gray's Anatomy for Students
   Drake RL, Vogl W, Mitchell AWM. *Gray's Anatomy for Students*. 4th ed. Elsevier.
3. Neuroanatomy Through Clinical Cases
   Blumenfeld H. *Neuroanatomy Through Clinical Cases*. 3rd ed. Sinauer Associates.
4. Principles of Neural Science
   Kandel ER, et al. *Principles of Neural Science*. 6th ed. McGraw-Hill.

Chapter 24

The Auditory Pathway: Anatomy, Physiology, Central Processing, and Clinical Correlates

Click here to view
Chapter Video: https://youtu.be/NEmbEibvRl0

Hearing begins when sound waves are collected by the external ear, mechanically amplified by the middle ear, and ultimately converted into neural signals within the inner ear. This process transforms mechanical vibrations into electrical impulses that are transmitted through a highly organized central pathway to the auditory cortex, where sound is perceived, interpreted, and integrated into meaningful experience. The auditory system thus bridges the physical properties of sound with higher cortical functions such as speech comprehension and environmental awareness.

The initial stages of sound processing involve conduction and amplification. The external ear acts as a funnel, directing sound waves toward the tympanic membrane. Vibrations of this membrane are transmitted through the ossicular chain of the middle ear—the malleus, incus, and stapes. This system functions as a mechanical lever, amplifying sound energy and efficiently transferring it from air to the fluid-filled inner ear. The footplate of the stapes rests on the oval window, through which mechanical energy is transmitted into the cochlea. To protect the delicate structures of the inner ear, an attenuation reflex is activated in response to loud sounds. This reflex involves contraction of the tensor tympani muscle, innervated by the trigeminal nerve, and the stapedius muscle, innervated by the facial nerve, thereby reducing ossicular movement and dampening sound transmission.

Within the inner ear, the cochlea serves as the primary organ of auditory transduction. This spiral-shaped bony structure encloses the cochlear duct, or scala media, which is filled with endolymph and flanked by the scala vestibuli and scala tympani, both containing perilymph. The oval window communicates with the scala vestibuli, allowing transmission of pressure waves, while the round window provides a flexible outlet for pressure dissipation within the scala tympani.

The organ of Corti, situated on the basilar membrane within the cochlear duct, contains the sensory apparatus for hearing. Inner hair cells function as the primary receptors, while outer hair cells amplify and fine-tune the mechanical vibrations of the basilar membrane. The stereocilia of these hair cells are embedded in the overlying tectorial membrane. When the stapes moves at the oval window, it generates pressure waves in the perilymph that propagate along the cochlea, displacing the basilar membrane. This displacement bends the stereocilia, leading to the opening of mechanically gated ion channels, depolarization of hair cells, and subsequent activation of spiral ganglion neurons. These neurons give rise to the cochlear division of the vestibulocochlear nerve, which carries auditory information into the brainstem.

A fundamental organizational principle of the auditory system is tonotopy, the spatial encoding of sound frequency. High-frequency sounds are detected at the base of the cochlea, near the oval window, whereas low-frequency sounds are detected at the apex. This orderly representation is preserved throughout the auditory pathway, from the cochlea to the cortex.

The central auditory pathway begins as the cochlear nerve enters the brainstem at the pontomedullary junction. Here, primary afferent fibers synapse in the dorsal and ventral cochlear nuclei. These nuclei represent the first level of central processing and give rise to multiple ascending pathways. A defining feature of the auditory system is its early bilateral representation; fibers from the cochlear nuclei project to both sides of the brain, which explains why unilateral lesions of higher auditory pathways rarely produce complete hearing loss.

One of the most important relay stations is the superior olivary complex in the pons, the first site at which input from both ears converges. This structure plays a critical role in sound localization by comparing interaural time differences and interaural intensity differences. These computations allow the brain to determine the direction from which a sound originates. From the superior olivary complex, ascending fibers form the lateral lemniscus, a prominent tract that carries auditory information to the midbrain.

The inferior colliculus, located in the midbrain, serves as a major integrative center for auditory processing. It is involved in sound localization, reflexive responses to auditory stimuli, and integration of binaural cues. From here, auditory signals are relayed to the medial geniculate nucleus of the thalamus, which acts as the principal thalamic relay for auditory information. The medial geniculate nucleus preserves the tonotopic organization established in the cochlea and transmits highly processed auditory signals to the cerebral cortex.

The primary auditory cortex, located in the transverse temporal gyrus (Heschl's gyrus) within the lateral sulcus, corresponds to Brodmann area 41. It receives precise, frequency-specific input and is responsible for the initial cortical processing of sound. Surrounding this region is the secondary auditory cortex, which further analyzes complex sound patterns. Beyond these areas lies the auditory association cortex, including regions such as Wernicke's area, which is essential for the comprehension of spoken language. Damage to this region results in Wernicke's aphasia, characterized by fluent but meaningless speech, impaired comprehension, and difficulty with repetition.

Clinically, disorders of the auditory system are broadly classified based on the level of impairment. Conductive hearing loss arises from abnormalities in the external or middle ear that impede sound transmission, such as tympanic membrane perforation, otitis media, or otosclerosis. In these conditions, air conduction is reduced while bone conduction remains relatively preserved.

Sensorineural hearing loss results from damage to the cochlea, hair cells, or auditory nerve. Common causes include prolonged noise exposure, ototoxic medications, age-related degeneration known as presbycusis, and inner ear disorders such as Ménière's disease. The latter is characterized by episodic vertigo, tinnitus, fluctuating hearing loss, and a sensation of aural fullness, resulting from endolymphatic hydrops within the cochlea.

Central auditory deficits are comparatively rare and typically require bilateral cortical involvement to produce significant hearing loss. Unilateral cortical lesions generally do not impair hearing but may disrupt sound localization and auditory discrimination. Lesions at the level of the cochlear nuclei, however, can produce unilateral hearing loss, often associated with lesions in the cerebellopontine angle, such as vestibular schwannomas.

In summary, the auditory pathway is a finely tuned and hierarchically organized system that converts mechanical sound waves into neural signals and integrates them into complex perceptual experiences. Its bilateral representation, tonotopic organization, and multiple relay stations allow for precise analysis of sound frequency, intensity, and spatial origin, enabling humans to perceive and interpret the rich auditory environment.

Review Questions

Q1. What structure contains the sensory receptors for hearing?
Answer: Organ of Corti.

Q2. Which hair cells are responsible for sound amplification?
Answer: Outer hair cells.

Q3. Where is the primary auditory cortex located?
Answer: Heschl's gyrus (BA 41).

Q4. What is the first site of binaural integration?
Answer: Superior olivary complex.

Q5. What type of hearing loss results from otosclerosis?
Answer: Conductive hearing loss.

Q6. What is preserved in conductive hearing loss?
Answer: Bone conduction.

Q7. What is the hallmark of Wernicke's aphasia?
Answer: Fluent but nonsensical speech with impaired comprehension.

Clinical Vignettes

Vignette 1 — Conductive Loss
A patient with chronic otitis media has reduced air conduction but normal bone conduction.
Diagnosis: Conductive hearing loss.

Vignette 2 — Sensorineural Loss
A factory worker with long-term exposure to noise presents with high-frequency hearing loss.
Diagnosis: Sensorineural hearing loss.

Vignette 3 — Cerebellopontine Angle Tumor
A patient presents with unilateral hearing loss and facial numbness.
Diagnosis: Vestibular schwannoma affecting the cochlear nucleus/nerve.

Vignette 4 — Wernicke's Aphasia
A patient speaks fluently but uses nonsensical words and cannot understand spoken language.
Diagnosis: Wernicke's aphasia (BA 22 lesion).

Vignette 5 — Ménière's Disease
A patient experiences episodic vertigo, tinnitus, and fluctuating hearing loss.
Diagnosis: Ménière's disease.

References

1. Neuroanatomy Through Clinical Cases
   Blumenfeld H. *Neuroanatomy Through Clinical Cases*. 3rd ed. Sinauer Associates.
2. Principles of Neural Science
   Kandel ER, et al. *Principles of Neural Science*. 6th ed. McGraw-Hill.
3. Ganong's Review of Medical Physiology
   Barrett KE, et al. *Ganong's Review of Medical Physiology*. 26th ed. McGraw-Hill.

Chapter 25

The Vestibular Pathway: Anatomy, Physiology, and Clinical Correlates

Click here to view
Chapter Video: https://youtu.be/PUBvcrLqKOY

Anatomy, Physiology, and Clinical Correlates

The vestibular system is the primary sensory apparatus responsible for equilibrium. It continuously provides information about head position, motion, and spatial orientation, thereby allowing the body to maintain balance, coordinate eye and head movements, and stabilize visual images during motion. In addition, it contributes to the subjective perception of movement, enabling an individual to sense acceleration, deceleration, and changes in position relative to gravity. Through extensive connections with the brainstem, cerebellum, spinal cord, and ocular motor nuclei, the vestibular system integrates sensory input with motor output to produce coordinated and adaptive responses.

The peripheral vestibular apparatus is located within the inner ear and consists of three semicircular canals and two otolith organs, the utricle and saccule. These structures are filled with endolymph, a potassium-rich fluid essential for the transduction of mechanical stimuli into neural signals. The semicircular canals are arranged in three orthogonal planes, allowing detection of rotational movements of the head in all spatial directions. The anterior canal is oriented to detect motion in the sagittal plane, the posterior canal in the coronal plane, and the lateral canal in the horizontal plane.

Each semicircular canal expands at one end into an ampulla, which contains the crista ampullaris, a specialized sensory epithelium. Within this structure, hair cells project their stereocilia into a gelatinous mass known as the cupula. During rotational head movement, inertia causes displacement of endolymph within the canal, leading to deflection of the cupula. This deflection bends the stereocilia of the hair cells, resulting in either depolarization or hyperpolarization depending on the direction of movement. These changes in membrane potential alter the firing rate of vestibular nerve fibers, thereby encoding angular acceleration.

In contrast to the semicircular canals, the otolith organs detect linear acceleration and gravitational forces. The utricle is primarily sensitive to horizontal linear acceleration, such as forward motion during rapid acceleration in a vehicle, whereas the saccule detects vertical acceleration, as experienced in an elevator, and also contributes to the perception of head position relative to gravity. Both organs contain a sensory region called the macula, composed of hair cells embedded in a gelatinous layer topped by otoliths, which are calcium carbonate crystals. These crystals increase the inertia of the system, enhancing sensitivity to linear acceleration. Movement of the head causes displacement of the otolithic membrane, bending the stereocilia and generating receptor potentials.

Disturbances in vestibular function often manifest as vertigo, a false sensation of movement typically described as spinning or whirling. This phenomenon arises when there is a mismatch between vestibular input and other sensory modalities, such as vision and proprioception. A common physiological example is the transient sensation of motion after stopping a spinning activity, due to continued movement of endolymph within the semicircular canals. Pathological causes of vertigo include vestibular neuritis, labyrinthitis, benign paroxysmal positional vertigo, Ménière's disease, and vestibular migraine. These conditions are frequently associated with nausea, vomiting, imbalance, and involuntary eye movements known as nystagmus.

Primary afferent neurons of the vestibular system have their cell bodies in the vestibular (Scarpa's) ganglion, located within the internal auditory canal. Their central processes enter the brainstem at the pontomedullary junction and synapse in the vestibular nuclear complex. This complex consists of four major nuclei: the superior, medial, lateral (Deiters'), and inferior vestibular nuclei. These nuclei serve as major integration centers, receiving input not only from the vestibular apparatus but also from the cerebellum, contralateral vestibular nuclei, visual pathways, and proprioceptive systems.

From the vestibular nuclei, multiple descending and ascending pathways distribute vestibular information throughout the nervous system. The vestibulospinal tracts are particularly important for postural control. The lateral vestibulospinal tract arises from the lateral vestibular nucleus and descends ipsilaterally throughout the spinal cord, facilitating extensor muscle tone and maintaining balance. The medial vestibulospinal tract originates from the medial vestibular nucleus and descends bilaterally to cervical and upper thoracic spinal levels, where it coordinates head and neck movements and contributes to the stabilization of gaze.

A critical functional component of the vestibular system is the vestibulo-ocular reflex (VOR), which ensures that visual images remain stable on the retina during head movement. This reflex operates through connections between the vestibular nuclei and the ocular motor nuclei of cranial nerves III, IV, and VI via the medial longitudinal fasciculus. When the head moves in one direction, the eyes move reflexively in the opposite direction, allowing fixation on a target. This response is rapid and automatic, and its integrity is essential for clear vision during motion.

The vestibular system is also closely integrated with the cerebellum, particularly the flocculonodular lobe, which is specialized for balance and eye–head coordination. Many vestibular afferents project directly to this region via the inferior cerebellar peduncle, while reciprocal connections between the cerebellum and vestibular nuclei form a feedback loop that refines postural control, gaze stabilization, and smooth pursuit eye movements.

Ascending vestibular pathways project to the thalamus, particularly the ventral posterior intermediate nucleus, and from there to cortical regions located in the insula and parietal lobe. These cortical areas are responsible for higher-order processing of vestibular information, including spatial orientation, perception of self-motion, and integration with visual and somatosensory inputs.

Clinically, vestibular dysfunction presents with characteristic signs and symptoms. Vertigo remains the most prominent feature, often accompanied by autonomic symptoms such as nausea and vomiting. Nystagmus, a rhythmic oscillation of the eyes, reflects an imbalance in vestibular input and provides important clues for the localization of lesions. Peripheral causes typically produce unidirectional nystagmus, whereas central causes may produce more complex patterns.

A notable disorder of the vestibular system is Ménière's disease, which is characterized by episodic vertigo, tinnitus, aural fullness, and fluctuating sensorineural hearing loss. The underlying mechanism involves endolymphatic hydrops, an abnormal accumulation of endolymph within the inner ear.

This condition illustrates the intimate relationship between auditory and vestibular function within the labyrinth.

In summary, the vestibular pathway represents a highly integrated sensory system that continuously monitors head motion and spatial orientation. Through its connections with motor, ocular, cerebellar, and cortical systems, it ensures stability of posture and gaze, enabling coordinated interaction with the environment. Its precise anatomical and functional organization allows clinicians to localize lesions based on characteristic patterns of vertigo, nystagmus, and postural disturbance.

Review Questions

Q1. Which vestibular structure detects horizontal linear acceleration?
Answer: Utricle.

Q2. What sensory structure detects angular acceleration?
Answer: Semicircular canals (crista ampullaris).

Q3. What is the function of the cupula?
Answer: Transmits endolymph movement to hair cell cilia.

Q4. Which vestibular nucleus gives rise to the lateral vestibulospinal tract?
Answer: Lateral vestibular nucleus (Deiters' nucleus).

Q5. What is the purpose of the vestibulo-ocular reflex?
Answer: Stabilizes gaze during head movement.

Q6. Which cerebellar lobe receives direct vestibular input?
Answer: Flocculonodular lobe.

Q7. What is the hallmark triad of Ménière's disease?
Answer: Vertigo, tinnitus, aural fullness.

Clinical Vignettes

Vignette 1 — BPPV

A patient experiences brief episodes of vertigo triggered by rolling over in bed. The Dix–Hallpike manoeuvre induces nystagmus.
Diagnosis: Benign paroxysmal positional vertigo (BPPV).

Vignette 2 — Vestibular Neuritis
A 40-year-old presents with acute vertigo, nausea, and vomiting, but no hearing loss.
Diagnosis: Vestibular neuritis (inflammation of the vestibular nerve).

Vignette 3 — Ménière's Disease
A patient reports episodic vertigo lasting hours, fluctuating hearing loss, and a sensation of fullness in the ear.
Diagnosis: Ménière's disease.

Vignette 4 — Central Vertigo
A patient with a cerebellar stroke presents with vertigo, severe gait ataxia, and direction-changing nystagmus.
Diagnosis: Central vestibular lesion.

Vignette 5 — VOR Testing
During rapid head rotation, a patient's eyes fail to maintain fixation.
Diagnosis: Impaired Vestibulo-ocular reflex (VOR).

References

1. Gray's Anatomy for Students
   Drake RL, Vogl W, Mitchell AWM. *Gray's Anatomy for Students*. 4th ed. Elsevier.
2. Neuroanatomy Through Clinical Cases
   Blumenfeld H. *Neuroanatomy Through Clinical Cases*. 3rd ed. Sinauer Associates.
3. Principles of Neural Science
   Kandel ER, et al. *Principles of Neural Science*. 6th ed. McGraw-Hill.

Chapter 26

Olfactory Pathways: Anatomy, Physiology, and Clinical Correlates

---

Click here to view
Chapter Video: https://youtu.be/lO-9x5XZjfA

The olfactory system consists of:

1. Olfactory epithelium
2. Olfactory nerves
3. Bulb and tract
4. Olfactory areas of the brain, collectively known as the rhinencephalon
5. Functional component: The olfactory nerve has only a special somatic afferent component.

The **olfactory system** is responsible for the special sense of smell and is one of the most primitive sensory systems in the brain, with strong connections to the limbic system.

It consists of four main components. First, the **olfactory epithelium**, located in the roof of the nasal cavity, contains specialized **olfactory receptor neurons**, which detect odorant molecules. Second, the **olfactory nerves**, also known as the fila olfactoria, are formed by the axons of these receptor neurons. These fibers pass through the **cribriform plate of the ethmoid bone** to reach the brain. Third, these fibers synapse in the **olfactory bulb**, which acts as the first relay station. The secondary neurons, particularly **mitral and tufted cells**, then project via the **olfactory tract** toward higher centers. Finally, the impulses reach the **olfactory cortical areas**, collectively referred to as the **rhinencephalon**, which include regions such as the piriform cortex, amygdala, and entorhinal cortex.

Functionally, the olfactory nerve is classified as a **special visceral afferent (SVA)** pathway, reflecting its role in detecting chemical stimuli related to smell. A unique and clinically important feature of the olfactory pathway is that it **bypasses the thalamus in its initial projection**, reaching the cortex directly. This distinguishes it from all other sensory systems and explains its strong association with **memory and emotional responses**. Thus, the olfactory pathway represents a direct link between the external chemical environment and higher cortical and limbic centers.

The **olfactory epithelium** is a specialized sensory epithelium located in the **roof of the nasal cavity**, including the **superior nasal concha and the upper part of the nasal septum**. This epithelium is maintained in a moist state by secretions from the **olfactory (Bowman's) glands**, which are essential for dissolving odorant molecules and facilitating their interaction with receptor cells. Histologically, the olfactory epithelium consists of three principal cell types. First, the **basal cells**, which function as **stem cells**. These cells continuously divide and give rise to new olfactory receptor neurons, making the olfactory system unique among sensory systems for its ability to undergo **regular neuronal regeneration**. Second, the **supporting cells**, also known as sustentacular cells, provide **structural and metabolic support** to the receptor neurons. Third, the **olfactory receptor neurons**, which are bipolar neurons responsible for detecting odorant molecules. These neurons extend dendrites to the epithelial surface and axons that form the olfactory nerve.

An important clinical point is that olfactory receptor neurons are **replaced approximately every 30 days**, reflecting ongoing turnover and regeneration.

This regenerative capacity is a distinctive feature of the olfactory system and has implications for recovery following injury or infection. Olfactory receptor neurons are specialized **bipolar neurons** located within the olfactory epithelium. Each neuron has a **peripherally directed dendrite** that ends in a bulbous expansion known as the **olfactory knob**. From this knob arise multiple **non-motile cilia**, which project into the mucus layer covering the epithelium. These cilia contain the **olfactory chemoreceptors**, where odorant molecules bind and initiate signal transduction. The **central processes (axons)** of these neurons form the **olfactory nerve filaments**, also known as the *fila olfactoria*. These numerous fine fibers, numbering in the millions, converge and pass through the **cribriform plate of the ethmoid bone**.

As they traverse this region, they organize into approximately **15 to 20 small bundles**, which collectively constitute the **olfactory nerve, or cranial nerve I**. These olfactory nerve fibers are ensheathed by specialized

glial cells, which provide structural support and play an important role in **axonal regeneration**. Notably, unlike most peripheral nerves, these fibers are **unmyelinated**, a feature relevant to their regenerative capacity. This unique organization allows continuous renewal of olfactory neurons while maintaining functional connectivity with the central nervous system.

Olfaction begins when **inhaled odorant molecules** dissolve in the **mucus layer** covering the olfactory epithelium. These molecules then bind to receptors located on the **cilia of olfactory receptor neurons**, initiating a cascade that generates **action potentials**.

These impulses are conducted along the **olfactory nerve filaments**, which pass through the **foramina of the cribriform plate** to enter the cranial cavity. As they ascend, these fibers traverse the meningeal layers and terminate in the **olfactory bulb**, which represents the first central relay station in the olfactory pathway. Within the olfactory bulb, the primary sensory neurons synapse with **second-order neurons**, mainly the **mitral cells and tufted cells**. These neurons are organized in distinct layers within the bulb. The incoming olfactory nerve fibers converge onto specialized synaptic structures known as **glomeruli**, where they form synapses with the dendrites of mitral and tufted cells.

In addition, the olfactory bulb contains **granule cells**, which are interneurons that modulate synaptic activity through inhibitory mechanisms, refining the olfactory signal. Thus, the olfactory bulb serves not only as a relay station but also as a site for **initial processing and integration of olfactory information** before it is transmitted to higher cortical centers.

The **mitral and tufted cells** of the olfactory bulb serve as the principal **second-order neurons**, transmitting olfactory information to higher cortical centers. Their axons form the **olfactory tract**, which carries processed olfactory signals posteriorly along the **inferior surface of the frontal lobe**, within the **olfactory sulcus**. An important feature is that some fibers, particularly from **tufted cells**, project to the **anterior olfactory nucleus**, which is located along the olfactory tract just posterior to the olfactory bulb. This nucleus plays a key role in **bilateral integration of olfactory information**, allowing communication between the two sides via commissural connections. Within the olfactory bulb, **granule cells** act as inhibitory interneurons, modulating the activity of mitral and tufted cells and refining odor discrimination. As the olfactory tract progresses posteriorly, it divides near the **anterior perforated substance** into two main pathways. The **medial olfactory stria** carries fibers that cross via the **anterior commissure** to the **contralateral olfactory bulb**, allowing bilateral integration of olfactory signals. The **lateral olfactory stria** is the major pathway and projects directly to the **primary olfactory cortex**, also known as the **piriform cortex.**

Thus, the olfactory tract serves as the major conduit for transmitting and integrating olfactory information before it reaches higher cortical and limbic regions.

The olfactory cortex can be functionally divided into **primary and secondary regions.** The **primary olfactory cortex** includes the **piriform cortex** and the **periamygdaloid cortex**, located primarily on the **ventromedial aspect of the temporal lobe**. This region receives direct input from the olfactory bulb and is unique among sensory systems in that it does **not require a thalamic relay** for initial cortical processing.

From the primary olfactory cortex, information is distributed to several important regions, including the **orbitofrontal cortex**, which is involved in conscious perception of smell; the **amygdala and hypothalamus**, which mediate emotional and autonomic responses; and the **entorhinal cortex and hippocampus**, which link olfaction to memory. Connections to the **insula** also contribute to integrative sensory processing. Clinically, the olfactory cortex, particularly the entorhinal region, is among the **earliest sites of degeneration in Alzheimer's disease**, which helps explain early symptoms such as impaired sense of smell. Thus, the olfactory pathway provides a direct and powerful link between sensory input and **emotion, behavior, and memory**.

The **secondary olfactory cortex** consists of higher-order cortical regions that further process and interpret olfactory information. These areas include the **uncus**, **orbitofrontal cortex**, **entorhinal cortex**, and the **amygdaloid complex**. Unlike the primary olfactory cortex, which receives direct input from the olfactory bulb, the secondary olfactory cortex is involved in the **conscious perception, integration, and emotional interpretation of odors.**

The **orbitofrontal cortex** plays a key role in the **conscious awareness and discrimination of smell**, allowing individuals to identify and differentiate specific odors. The **amygdala** is involved in the **affective and emotional aspects of olfaction**, determining whether an odor is perceived as pleasant or unpleasant, and linking it to behavioral responses. The **entorhinal cortex** serves as an interface with the hippocampus, facilitating the association of odors with **memory and experience**. The **uncus**, part of the medial temporal lobe, is closely related to olfactory processing and is clinically significant, as lesions or seizures in this region may produce **olfactory hallucinations,** known as uncinate fits. Thus, the secondary olfactory cortex integrates sensory input with **perception, emotion, and memory**, completing the olfactory processing pathway.

Olfactory disorders are clinically important and may help localize lesions along the olfactory pathway. **Anosmia** refers to the **complete loss of the sense of smell**, whereas **hyposmia** indicates a **reduced ability to perceive odors**. These conditions most commonly result from damage to the **olfactory receptor neurons or olfactory nerve fibers**, such as after viral infections or trauma. **Dyssomnia**, also termed parosmia, refers to a **distorted perception of smell** and is often associated with **cortical or central pathway dysfunction**, including lesions affecting higher olfactory centers.

Bilateral anosmia is most commonly due to **inflammation of the nasal mucosa**, which interferes with odorant access to the olfactory epithelium. Common causes include the **common cold, allergic rhinitis, and atrophic rhinitis.**

In contrast, **unilateral anosmia** usually indicates a lesion along the olfactory pathway on one side, such as involvement of the **olfactory nerve, olfactory bulb, or olfactory tract**, particularly **proximal to its bifurcation.** Thus, careful assessment of olfactory dysfunction can provide valuable clues for **localizing pathology** within the peripheral or central components of the olfactory system.

Olfactory abnormalities can arise from both **peripheral** and **central causes and** distinguishing between these is important for clinical localization. **Peripheral causes** affect the olfactory epithelium or the access of odorants to receptor neurons. Common examples include **upper respiratory infections**, which can damage the olfactory mucosa; **nasal obstruction**, such as from polyps or inflammation, which prevents odorants from reaching the receptors; and certain **medications**, which may alter olfactory function.

In contrast, **central causes** involve pathology along the olfactory pathway beyond the epithelium. These include **neuronal dysfunction affecting the olfactory nerve, bulb, or tract**, as well as **head injury**, which may shear the olfactory nerve fibers at the cribriform plate. Olfactory dysfunction is also commonly associated with **aging** and **neurodegenerative diseases**, where it may serve as an early clinical sign. In addition, certain **psychiatric disorders** may alter the perception of smell.

Thus, evaluation of olfactory abnormalities requires consideration of both peripheral and central mechanisms to accurately identify the underlying cause.

Review Questions

Q1 A 30-year-old man presents with loss of smell following a head injury. Which structure is most likely damaged?

A. Olfactory bulb
B. Cribriform plate
C. Optic chiasm
D. Superior colliculus
E. Internal capsule

Answer: B. Cribriform plate

Explanation: Trauma can shear **olfactory nerve filaments** as they pass through the **cribriform plate**, leading to anosmia.

Q2 Which of the following is a unique feature of the olfactory pathway compared to other sensory systems?

A. Bilateral cortical representation
B. Direct projection to cortex without thalamic relay
C. Synapse in the medulla
D. Crossing at the spinal cord level
E. Use of lower motor neurons

Answer: B. Direct projection to cortex without thalamic relay

Explanation: The olfactory pathway is unique in that it bypasses the thalamus initially and projects directly to the primary olfactory cortex.

Q3 Olfactory receptor neurons are continuously replaced by which of the following cell types?

A. Mitral cells
B. Tufted cells
C. Granule cells
D. Basal cells
E. Schwann cells

Answer: D. Basal cells

Explanation: **Basal cells** act as stem cells and regenerate olfactory receptor neurons approximately every 30 days.

Q.4 A patient reports perceiving foul odors that are not present. This is most likely due to a lesion in which region?

A. Nasal septum
B. Olfactory epithelium
C. Primary olfactory cortex

D. Occipital lobe
E. Cerebellum

Answer: C. Primary olfactory cortex

Explanation: Distorted smell perception **(dyssomnia/parosmia)** is often due to **cortical lesions**, particularly in olfactory cortical areas.

Q.5 Which structure is primarily responsible for the emotional response to odors?

A. Orbitofrontal cortex
B. Amygdala
C. Hippocampus
D. Thalamus
E. Insula

Answer: B. Amygdala

Explanation: The **amygdala** mediates the **affective and emotional components** of olfactory stimuli.

References

1. **Snell RS.** *Clinical Neuroanatomy*, 8th/9th Edition. Wolters Kluwer.
2. **Blumenfeld H.** *Neuroanatomy through Clinical Cases*, 3rd Edition. Sinauer/Oxford.
3. **Kandel ER, et al.** *Principles of Neural Science*, 6th Edition. McGraw-Hill.
4. **Standring S (Ed.).** *Gray's Anatomy: The Anatomical Basis of Clinical Practice*, 42nd Edition. Elsevier.
5. **Guyton & Hall.** *Textbook of Medical Physiology*, 14th Edition. Elsevier.

Chapter 27

Cranial Nerves - 3 to 7 (Only video presentation- no Textual description appended)

Click here to view
Chapter Video: https://youtu.be/f9wuIxio-iU

Chapter 28

Cranial Nerves - 9 to 12 (Only video presentation - No textual description appended)

Click here to view
Chapter Video: https://youtu.be/qKkgvg3dfyQ

Chapter 29

Internal Capsule: Anatomy, Fiber Composition, Blood Supply, and Stroke Syndromes

---

Click here to view
Chapter Video: https://youtu.be/0pTboInnzKg

The internal capsule is one of the most critical white matter structures of the brain, serving as the principal conduit through which ascending sensory information and descending motor commands pass between the cerebral cortex, brainstem, and spinal cord. Its functional importance is magnified by its compact organization, in which a vast number of fibers are tightly packed within a relatively small anatomical space. Consequently, even a small lesion in this region can result in profound and often devastating neurological deficits. A precise understanding of its anatomy, fiber composition, and vascular supply is therefore essential for accurate clinical localization, particularly in the context of cerebrovascular disease.

Anatomically, the internal capsule is situated deep within the cerebral hemispheres and forms a V-shaped band of white matter interposed between major components of the basal ganglia. The anterior limb lies between the head of the caudate nucleus medially and the lentiform nucleus laterally. At the junction of the anterior and posterior limbs is the genu, which represents the bend of the capsule. The posterior limb is positioned between the thalamus medially and the lentiform nucleus laterally. Superiorly, the fibers of the internal capsule diverge into the corona radiata, spreading widely toward the cerebral cortex. Inferiorly, they converge to form the cerebral peduncles of the midbrain. Additional components include the retrolentiform part, which passes posterior to the lentiform nucleus, and the Sublentiform part, which passes inferior to it. Together, these segments create a structural framework that "encapsulates" the lentiform nucleus internally, complementing the external capsule that lies lateral to it.

The internal capsule is classically divided into five anatomical parts: the anterior limb, genu, posterior limb, retrolentiform part, and Sublentiform part. Each segment contains distinct fiber systems with specific functional roles.

The anterior limb contains frontopontine fibers, which connect the frontal cortex to the pons, as well as thalamocortical and corticothalamic fibers linking the frontal lobe with anterior and dorsomedial thalamic nuclei. These connections are involved in executive function, behavioral regulation, and limbic integration.

The genu contains corticobulbar, or corticonuclear, fibers that project to the motor nuclei of cranial nerves in the brainstem. This region marks the beginning of somatotopic organization within the internal capsule, with fibers representing the face located most anteriorly. As one moves posteriorly into the posterior limb, this somatotopic arrangement continues in an orderly fashion, with fibers representing the arm, trunk, and leg arranged sequentially.

The posterior limb is the most functionally significant portion of the internal capsule. It contains corticospinal fibers responsible for voluntary motor control, as well as superior thalamic radiations that convey somatosensory information from the ventral posterior nuclei of the thalamus to the primary somatosensory cortex. Notably, motor and sensory fibers are spatially segregated within this region, which explains the sharply defined clinical deficits observed in lesions affecting the posterior limb.

The retrolentiform part contains the optic radiation, also known as geniculocalcarine fibers, which transmit visual information from the lateral geniculate nucleus to the primary visual cortex. It also contains parietopontine fibers and posterior thalamic radiations. Lesions in this region typically produce contralateral homonymous hemianopia.

The Sublentiform part contains the auditory radiation, which connects the medial geniculate nucleus to the superior temporal gyrus, as well as temporopontine fibers. Damage to this region may result in auditory deficits or, in the dominant hemisphere, disturbances of language comprehension resembling Wernicke-type aphasia.

The vascular supply of the internal capsule is derived from small, penetrating arteries that arise primarily from major cerebral vessels. These arteries are end-arterial in nature, meaning they lack significant collateral circulation, rendering the internal capsule particularly vulnerable to ischemic injury. The anterior limb is supplied by medial striate arteries, including the recurrent artery of Heubner from the anterior cerebral artery, as well as lateral lenticulostriate branches of the middle cerebral artery. The genu is primarily supplied by lateral lenticulostriate arteries, with occasional contributions from branches of the internal carotid artery or the anterior choroidal artery. The posterior limb receives its principal blood supply from the anterior choroidal artery, a branch of the internal carotid artery, with additional input from lenticulostriate arteries. The retrolentiform and Sublentiform parts are also predominantly supplied by the anterior choroidal artery.

Because these vessels are small and subject to pathological changes such as lipohyalinosis, particularly in chronic hypertension, they are common sites of lacunar infarction. Occlusion of these arteries produces sharply demarcated lesions with predictable clinical manifestations.

Stroke syndromes involving the internal capsule are characterized by deficits that reflect the specific fiber tracts affected. Importantly, cortical signs such as aphasia, neglect, or higher visual deficits are typically absent, which helps distinguish capsular lesions from cortical strokes. Infarction of the posterior limb is the most common and clinically significant presentation. It produces contralateral hemiparesis involving the face, arm, and leg, often accompanied by contralateral hemisensory loss if thalamic radiations are involved. This presentation is the classic example of a pure motor or sensorimotor lacunar stroke.

Lesions involving the genu primarily affect corticobulbar fibers and result in contralateral lower facial weakness, dysarthria, and occasionally deviation of the tongue or uvula due to involvement of cranial nerve motor pathways. Infarction of the anterior limb tends to produce more subtle deficits, including executive dysfunction, apathy, or abulia, reflecting disruption of frontal–thalamic circuits, along with mild contralateral weakness.

Damage to the retrolentiform portion leads to visual field defects, most notably contralateral homonymous hemianopia due to involvement of the optic radiation. Lesions of the Sublentiform portion may impair auditory processing and, in the dominant hemisphere, produce receptive language deficits resembling Wernicke's aphasia.

In summary, the internal capsule represents a compact and highly organized hub through which essential motor and sensory pathways pass. Its strategic location and dense fiber composition make it particularly susceptible to small but clinically significant vascular lesions. The precise pattern of neurological deficits resulting from such lesions provides valuable insight into the underlying neuroanatomy and remains a cornerstone of clinical localization in neurology.

Clinical Vignette

A 62-year-old man with hypertension suddenly develops weakness of the right face, arm, and leg. He is alert, oriented, and has no aphasia, no visual field deficits, and no neglect. MRI shows a small infarct in the left posterior limb of the internal capsule.

Diagnosis: Lacunar infarct of the posterior limb due to occlusion of a lateral lenticulostriate artery.
Explanation: The tightly packed corticospinal fibers in the posterior limb produce a pure motor stroke when damaged. The absence of cortical signs localizes the lesion to the internal capsule rather than the cortex.

Review Questions

Q1. Which artery most commonly supplies the posterior limb of the internal capsule?
Answer: Anterior choroidal artery.

Q2. Which fibers are located in the genu of the internal capsule?
Answer: Corticobulbar (corticonuclear) fibers.

Q3. A lesion of the retrolentiform part of the internal capsule produces which deficit?
Answer: Contralateral homonymous hemianopia.

Q4. What is the classic clinical presentation of a lacunar infarct in the posterior limb?
Answer: Pure motor hemiparesis.

Q5. Which part of the internal capsule carries auditory radiations?
Answer: Sublentiform part.

References

1. Kandel, E. R., Schwartz, J. H., Jessell, T. M., et al. *Principles of Neural Science*. McGraw-Hill.
2. DeLong, M. R., & Wichmann, T. Basal ganglia circuits and movement disorders. *JAMA Neurology*.

3. Lanciego, J. L., Luquin, N., & Obeso, J. A. Functional neuroanatomy of the basal ganglia. *Progress in Neurobiology.*
4. Obeso, J. A., Stamelou, M., Goetz, C. G., et al. Past, present, and future of Parkinson's disease. *Lancet Neurology.*
5. Albin, R. L., Young, A. B., & Penney, J. B. The functional anatomy of basal ganglia disorders. *Trends in Neurosciences.*

Chapter 30

Neuropsychology and Behavior: Brain Circuits, Functional Networks, and Clinical Correlates

Click here to view
Chapter Video: https://youtu.be/L3tS86STjVE

Brain Circuits, Functional Networks, and Clinical Correlates

Psychiatric disorders are no longer understood as the consequence of isolated lesions in discrete brain regions. Instead, modern neuroscience conceptualizes them as disorders of distributed neural systems, arising from complex interactions among genetic predisposition, environmental influences, and neurobiological processes. These conditions reflect dysfunction in interconnected brain circuits and large-scale functional networks that regulate cognition, emotion, motivation, and behavior. Alterations in connectivity, neurotransmitter dynamics, and network activity patterns form the basis of most psychiatric syndromes.

At the regional level, several key brain structures play central roles in the pathophysiology of psychiatric disorders. The prefrontal cortex serves as the executive center of the brain, governing decision-making, working memory, impulse control, and emotional regulation. Dysfunction in this region, often described as Hypofrontality, is a hallmark of conditions such as schizophrenia, major depressive disorder, attention-deficit/hyperactivity disorder, and bipolar disorder. This is frequently accompanied by reduced Gray matter volume and impaired connectivity with limbic structures, particularly the amygdala and hippocampus.

The amygdala is critical for emotional processing, especially fear and threat detection. In anxiety disorders and post-traumatic stress disorder, it often exhibits hyperactivity, reflecting heightened emotional reactivity.

Disrupted connectivity between the amygdala and prefrontal cortex further impairs the regulation of emotional responses. The hippocampus, essential for memory consolidation and contextual processing, is particularly vulnerable to chronic stress. Many psychiatric conditions, including depression and PTSD, are associated with reduced hippocampal volume, impaired synaptic plasticity, and decreased neurogenesis.

The anterior cingulate cortex plays an integrative role in emotional regulation, error detection, and conflict monitoring. Abnormal activation and altered connectivity of this region are observed in depression, obsessive-compulsive disorder, and bipolar disorder. Similarly, the basal ganglia, traditionally associated with motor control, are now recognized for their role in habit formation and reward processing. Dysregulation of dopaminergic pathways within cortico-striato-thalamo-cortical circuits contributes to disorders such as OCD, Tourette syndrome, and schizophrenia.

The thalamus functions as a central relay station, integrating and modulating sensory and cortical information. In psychiatric disorders, particularly schizophrenia and bipolar disorder, thalamocortical connectivity is often disrupted, leading to impaired sensory gating and altered conscious experience.

Beyond individual regions, psychiatric disorders are best understood through the lens of large-scale brain networks. The default mode network is active during rest and is involved in self-referential thinking, introspection, and memory retrieval. In depression, this network often shows hyperconnectivity, contributing to persistent rumination. In contrast, reduced connectivity within this network is observed in attention-deficit/hyperactivity disorder, while disrupted coherence is characteristic of autism spectrum disorders.

The central executive network is responsible for goal-directed behavior, working memory, and cognitive flexibility. It involves the dorsolateral prefrontal cortex, anterior cingulate cortex, and parietal regions. Dysfunction in this network manifests as impaired task performance and reduced cognitive control in disorders such as schizophrenia, depression, and dementia.

The salience network plays a pivotal role in identifying behaviorally relevant stimuli and mediating the dynamic switching between the default mode and central executive networks. It integrates emotional and sensory inputs to guide attention and behavior. Abnormal salience attribution, as seen in schizophrenia, may underlie hallucinations and delusions, while impaired network switching contributes to cognitive and emotional dysregulation in several psychiatric conditions.

Genetic and neurochemical factors further shape the neurobiology of psychiatric disorders. Most conditions exhibit polygenic inheritance, with multiple genes interacting with environmental influences. Neurotransmitter systems are critically involved: serotonin regulates mood and anxiety; dopamine is central to reward processing, psychosis, and attention; norepinephrine modulates arousal and stress responses; gamma-aminobutyric acid provides inhibitory control; and glutamate mediates excitatory transmission and synaptic plasticity. Imbalances in these systems contribute to the diverse clinical manifestations of psychiatric illness.

Major psychiatric disorders can be understood within this integrated framework. Depression is characterized by persistent low mood, anhedonia, and cognitive slowing, associated with monoamine deficiencies, hippocampal atrophy, and hyperactivity of the default mode network. Anxiety disorders involve excessive fear and autonomic arousal, driven by amygdala hyperactivity and reduced prefrontal inhibition. Autism spectrum disorder reflects abnormalities in network connectivity, particularly within the default mode network, along with disruptions in neurotransmitter systems and social processing circuits.

Attention-deficit/hyperactivity disorder arises from dysfunction in frontostriatal circuits, leading to impaired executive function and reduced dopaminergic and noradrenergic signaling. Obsessive-compulsive disorder is associated with hyperactivity in orbitofrontal and anterior cingulate circuits, along with imbalances in glutamate and GABA neurotransmission. Schizophrenia involves widespread dysconnectivity, particularly within thalamocortical circuits, along with disturbances in dopamine, serotonin, and glutamate systems, resulting in psychosis and cognitive impairment. Bipolar disorder reflects instability in limbic–prefrontal circuits and altered reward processing, producing alternating episodes of mania and depression.

In summary, neuropsychology and behavior are governed by highly integrated and dynamic brain systems. Psychiatric disorders emerge from disruptions at multiple levels, including regional dysfunction, circuit abnormalities, network dysregulation, and neurochemical imbalance. This systems-based perspective provides a more comprehensive understanding of mental illness and underpins modern approaches to diagnosis, treatment, and research.

Summary Sheet

Psychiatric disorders arise from interactions among genetic, environmental, and neurobiological factors. Modern neuroscience shows that these conditions reflect dysfunction in specific brain regions, distributed neural circuits, and largescale functional networks that regulate emotion, cognition, motivation, and behavior.

1. Key Brain Regions Involved in Psychiatric Disorders

Prefrontal Cortex (PFC)

- Functions: executive function, decisionmaking, impulse control
- Disorders: schizophrenia, depression, ADHD, bipolar disorder
- Findings: Hypofrontality, reduced grey matter, impaired connectivity with limbic regions

Amygdala

- Functions: emotional processing, fear response
- Disorders: anxiety disorders, PTSD, schizophrenia
- Findings: volume changes, hyperactivity, dysregulated amygdala–PFC connectivity

Hippocampus

- Functions: memory consolidation, stress regulation
- Disorders: depression, PTSD, schizophrenia
- Findings: reduced neurogenesis, impaired plasticity, volume loss

Anterior Cingulate Cortex (ACC)

- Functions: error detection, emotional regulation
- Disorders: depression, OCD, bipolar disorder
- Findings: abnormal activation, altered limbic–frontal connectivity

Basal Ganglia

- Functions: motor control, habit formation, reward processing
- Disorders: OCD, Tourette syndrome, schizophrenia

Findings: structural abnormalities, dopaminergic dysregulation

Thalamus

- Functions: sensory relay, consciousness, information integration
- Disorders: schizophrenia, bipolar disorder
- Findings: volume reduction, disrupted thalamocortical connectivity

2. **Large-Scale Brain Networks**

Psychiatric disorders reflect dysfunction in distributed networks, not isolated regions.

Default Mode Network (DMN)

- Functions: self-referential thought, introspection, memory retrieval
- Regions: medial PFC, posterior cingulate, precuneus, angular gyrus
- Disorders: depression, anxiety, ADHD, autism
- Findings: hyperconnectivity (rumination), hypoconnectivity (ADHD)

Central Executive Network (CEN)

- Functions: working memory, problemsolving, planning, cognitive flexibility
- Regions: dorsolateral PFC, ACC, orbitofrontal cortex, inferior parietal lobule
- Disorders: depression, schizophrenia, autism, PTSD, dementia
- Findings: impaired activation, reduced connectivity

Salience Network (SN)

- Functions: detecting relevant stimuli, switching between DMN and CEN
- Regions: anterior insula, dorsal ACC, amygdala, ventral striatum
- Disorders: anxiety, autism, schizophrenia, bipolar disorder
- Findings: abnormal salience attribution, impaired network switching

3. **Neurochemical and Genetic Contributions**

Key Neurotransmitters

- Serotonin → mood, anxiety, impulsivity
- Dopamine → reward, psychosis, attention
- Norepinephrine → arousal, stress response
- GABA → inhibition, anxiety regulation
- Glutamate → excitatory signaling, plasticity

Genetics

- Many disorders are polygenic
- Strong familial clustering in autism, ADHD, bipolar disorder, schizophrenia, depression

4. Overview of Major Psychiatric Disorders

Depression

- Low mood, anhedonia
- Reduced monoamines (5HT, NE, dopamine)
- Hyperactive DMN, reduced hippocampal neurogenesis
- Treated with antidepressants and psychotherapy

Anxiety Disorders

- Excessive fear, autonomic hyperarousal
- Amygdala hyperactivity, reduced PFC inhibition
- Involves serotonin, norepinephrine, and GABA
- Treated with SSRIs/SNRIs, CBT

Autism Spectrum Disorder

- Social and communication deficits
- DMN abnormalities, GABA/serotonin imbalance
- Calcium signaling dysregulation
- Genetic contributions significant but not deterministic

ADHD

- Inattention, impulsivity, hyperactivity
- Dysfunction of frontostriatal circuits
- Low dopamine and norepinephrine
- Impaired executive function

ObsessiveCompulsive Disorder (OCD)

- Intrusive thoughts, compulsive behaviors
- Hyperactive orbitofrontal cortex and ACC
- Increased putamen/globus pallidus volume
- Glutamate/GABA imbalance

Schizophrenia

- Delusions, hallucinations, disorganized thought
- Dopamine, serotonin, glutamate imbalance
- Thalamocortical dysconnectivity
- Genetic predisposition is significant

Bipolar Disorder

- Alternating mania and depression
- Dysregulated limbic–prefrontal circuits
- Abnormal reward processing
- Polygenic inheritance

Review Questions

Q1. Which brain region shows Hypofrontality in schizophrenia?
Answer: Prefrontal cortex.

Q2. Which network is hyperactive in depressive rumination?
Answer: Default Mode Network (DMN).

Q3. Which neurotransmitter is most associated with reward and psychosis?
Answer: Dopamine.

Q4. Which structure is central to fear processing?
Answer: Amygdala.

Q5. Which disorder involves dysfunction of the frontostriatal network?
Answer: ADHD.

Q6. Which psychiatric disorder shows increased activity in the orbitofrontal cortex and ACC?
Answer: ObsessiveCompulsive Disorder (OCD).

Q7. Which cortical region is essential for speech comprehension and is affected in schizophrenia?
Answer: Wernicke's area (BA 22).

Q8. Which neurotransmitter system is most implicated in depression?
Answer: Serotonin (also norepinephrine, dopamine).

Q9. What brain region shows hyperactivity in anxiety disorders?
Answer: Amygdala.

Q10. Which pathway is hyperactive in schizophrenia, producing positive symptoms?
Answer: Mesolimbic dopamine pathway.

Q11. OCD is associated with hyperactivity in which circuit?
Answer: Orbitofrontal–striatal circuit.

Q12. What structural change is often seen in chronic depression?
Answer: Hippocampal atrophy.

Clinical Vignettes

Vignette 1 — Depression
A patient presents with persistent low mood, anhedonia, and impaired concentration. MRI shows reduced hippocampal volume.
Diagnosis: Major depressive disorder.

Vignette 2 — PTSD
A veteran experiences flashbacks and hypervigilance. fMRI shows amygdala hyperactivity and reduced PFC inhibition.
Diagnosis: Post-traumatic stress disorder.

Vignette 3 — Autism
A child has difficulty with social interaction and face recognition. Imaging shows DMN abnormalities.
Diagnosis: Autism spectrum disorder.

Vignette 4 — OCD
A patient reports intrusive thoughts and repetitive handwashing. Imaging shows hyperactivity in the orbitofrontal cortex.
Diagnosis: Obsessive-compulsive disorder.

Vignette 5 — Schizophrenia
A young adult presents with auditory hallucinations and disorganized speech. Imaging reveals thalamocortical dysconnectivity.
Diagnosis: Schizophrenia.

References

1. Kandel, E. R., Schwartz, J. H., Jessell, T. M., et al. *Principles of Neural Science.* McGraw-Hill.
2. DeLong, M. R., & Wichmann, T. Basal ganglia circuits and movement disorders. *JAMA Neurology.*
3. Lanciego, J. L., Luquin, N., & Obeso, J. A. Functional neuroanatomy of the basal ganglia. *Progress in Neurobiology.*
4. Obeso, J. A., Stamelou, M., Goetz, C. G., et al. Past, present, and future of Parkinson's disease. *Lancet Neurology.*
5. Albin, R. L., Young, A. B., & Penney, J. B. The functional anatomy of basal ganglia disorders. *Trends in Neurosciences.*

Chapter 31

Basal Ganglia: Organization, Components, and Functional Architecture

Click here to view
Chapter Video: https://youtu.be/5eLT-C4AdSg

Hierarchical Context of Motor Control

Motor control within the human nervous system is organized in a hierarchical manner, with multiple levels contributing to the planning, modulation, and execution of movement. At the highest level, the motor cortex initiates voluntary movement. The brainstem regulates posture, tone, and reflexive motor activity, while the spinal cord serves as the final common pathway through which motor commands are executed via lower motor neurons. Interposed between these levels are the basal ganglia and cerebellum, which function as parallel modulatory systems that refine and optimize motor output. Before any voluntary movement is executed, it is first conceptualized, planned, and programmed within the premotor and supplementary motor areas. These preparatory processes are then transmitted to the primary motor cortex, which integrates essential feedback from the basal ganglia and cerebellum to ensure that movement is precise, coordinated, and appropriately scaled.

The basal ganglia play a central role in the selection and control of motor programs. Their primary function is not the initiation of movement per se, but rather the facilitation of intended movements and the suppression of competing or unwanted motor activity. In addition, they regulate the amplitude and velocity of movement, contributing to smooth and purposeful motor execution. This is particularly evident in skilled tasks such as writing or fine object manipulation, where precise coordination between agonist and antagonist muscle groups is required. Dysfunction of the basal ganglia leads to characteristic movement disorders. Reduced facilitation of motor activity results in hypokinetic states, as seen in Parkinsonian syndromes, whereas failure to suppress unwanted movements produces hyperkinetic disorders such as chorea and ballismus. Thus, the basal ganglia are indispensable for the initiation, scaling, and refinement of voluntary movement.

Anatomically, the basal ganglia consist of a group of interconnected nuclei located within the cerebral hemispheres, diencephalon, and midbrain. These include the caudate nucleus, putamen, globus pallidus, subthalamic nucleus, and substantia nigra. The globus pallidus is divided into external (GPe) and internal (GPi) segments, while the substantia nigra is subdivided into the pars compacta (SNc) and pars reticulata (SNr). Functionally, the caudate nucleus and putamen together form the striatum, which serves as the principal input structure of the basal ganglia. Although these two structures are separated by the anterior limb of the internal capsule, they remain functionally unified and exhibit a characteristic striated appearance due to interspersed fiber bundles.

At the ventral junction of the caudate and putamen lies the nucleus accumbens, which forms the ventral striatum. This region is critically involved in motivation, reward processing, reinforcement learning, and the integration of emotional states with goal-directed behavior. The globus pallidus, particularly its internal segment, along with the substantia nigra pars reticulata, constitutes the major output system of the basal ganglia, projecting to the thalamus and brainstem motor centers.

The subthalamic nucleus occupies a key position within the basal ganglia circuitry, lying ventral to the thalamus. It plays an essential role in the indirect pathway, which suppresses unwanted movement. Lesions of this nucleus result in hemiballismus, a disorder characterized by violent, flinging movements of the contralateral limbs, reflecting a loss of inhibitory control over thalamocortical motor output. The substantia nigra, located in the midbrain, is notable for its pigmented dopaminergic neurons. The pars compacta provides dopaminergic input to the striatum, while the pars reticulata functions analogously to the GPi as an output nucleus. Degeneration of dopaminergic neurons in the pars compacta underlies Parkinson's disease, producing bradykinesia, rigidity, and resting tremor. Dopamine exerts its effects through D1 receptors, which facilitate the direct pathway, and D2 receptors, which inhibit the indirect pathway, thereby promoting movement initiation.

The thalamus serves as a critical relay station in basal ganglia circuits, particularly through the ventral anterior and ventral lateral nuclei, which project to the motor cortex. The basal ganglia receive extensive input from multiple cortical and subcortical regions, including the motor, premotor, and somatosensory cortices, as well as limbic structures such as the amygdala. Additional modulatory input arises from brainstem nuclei, including dopaminergic projections from the substantia nigra, serotonergic input from the raphe nuclei, and noradrenergic input from the locus coeruleus. Within the striatum, local interneurons, including cholinergic neurons, further modulate synaptic activity and influence the balance between excitatory and inhibitory pathways.

Functionally, the basal ganglia operate through two principal circuits: the direct and indirect pathways. These pathways form a dynamic balance that regulates motor output through a series of excitatory and inhibitory interactions. The direct pathway facilitates movement by reducing inhibitory output from the GPi to the thalamus. When the striatum inhibits the GPi, the thalamus is disinhibited, allowing it to activate the motor cortex and promote movement. In contrast, the indirect pathway suppresses unwanted movement by increasing inhibitory output to the thalamus. In this pathway, inhibition of the external segment of the globus pallidus leads to activation of the subthalamic nucleus, which in turn excites the GPi, resulting in enhanced inhibition of thalamocortical activity.

Dopamine plays a pivotal modulatory role in these circuits by simultaneously enhancing the direct pathway and suppressing the indirect pathway, thereby facilitating movement. The precise balance between these pathways ensures that intended movements are executed smoothly while competing motor programs are suppressed. Disruption of this balance leads to either excessive inhibition of the thalamus, resulting in hypokinesia, or insufficient inhibition, resulting in hyperkinesia.

Clinically, disorders of the basal ganglia are broadly classified into hypokinetic and hyperkinetic syndromes. Parkinson's disease represents the prototypical hypokinetic disorder and results from degeneration of dopaminergic neurons in the substantia nigra pars compacta. This leads to decreased activation of the direct pathway and increased activity of the indirect pathway, culminating in reduced thalamocortical stimulation. Pathologically, Parkinson's disease is characterized by the presence of Lewy bodies, composed primarily of alpha-synuclein, within affected neurons. Advances in diagnostic techniques now include alpha-synuclein seed amplification assays and functional imaging such as dopamine transporter scans, which aid in distinguishing Parkinson's disease from other movement disorders. Treatment strategies focus on restoring dopaminergic function through agents such as levodopa combined with carbidopa, dopamine agonists, monoamine oxidase-B inhibitors, and catechol-O-methyltransferase inhibitors. In advanced cases, deep brain stimulation targeting the subthalamic nucleus or globus pallidus internus provides significant symptomatic relief.

Hyperkinetic disorders arise from reduced inhibitory output of the basal ganglia, leading to excessive cortical excitation. These include a spectrum of abnormal movements such as tremor, dystonia, chorea, athetosis, myoclonus, and ballismus. Tourette syndrome, characterized by motor and vocal tics, represents a disorder of basal ganglia circuitry with onset typically in childhood. Management includes behavioral therapy, pharmacological agents such as alpha-2 agonists and antipsychotics, and, in severe cases, deep brain stimulation. Myoclonus, defined by sudden, brief, involuntary muscle jerks, may arise from a variety of physiological or pathological conditions and reflects dysfunction at multiple levels of the motor system.

In summary, the basal ganglia constitute a complex network of interconnected nuclei that regulate motor function through finely balanced excitatory and inhibitory pathways. By facilitating desired movements and suppressing unwanted activity, they ensure that motor behavior is smooth, coordinated, and adaptive. Their dysfunction gives rise to a wide range of movement disorders, underscoring their critical role in human motor control.

Summary Sheet

The basal ganglia are interconnected subcortical nuclei that regulate the initiation, scaling, and suppression of movement. They function as a major sideloop in the motor hierarchy, refining cortical motor programs and ensuring smooth, coordinated, and purposeful activity. Their influence extends beyond motor control to include motivation, reward, habit formation, and emotional modulation.

Major Components

- Striatum: caudate nucleus, putamen
- Globus pallidus: external (GPe) and internal (GPi) segments
- Subthalamic nucleus (STN)
- Substantia nigra: pars compacta (SNc), pars reticulata (SNr)
- Nucleus accumbens (ventral striatum)

Functional Organization

- Direct pathway → facilitates movement
- Indirect pathway → suppresses unwanted movement
- Dopamine (SNc):
    - Excites D1 neurons (direct pathway)
    - Inhibits D2 neurons (indirect pathway)
- Net effect of dopamine: promotes movement

Direct Pathway (Movement Facilitation)

1. D1 striatal neurons inhibit GPi
2. GPi reduces the inhibition of the thalamus
3. The thalamus excites the motor cortex
4. Movement is initiated or sustained

Indirect Pathway (Movement Suppression)

1. D2 striatal neurons inhibit GPe
2. GPe reduces the inhibition of STN
3. STN excites GPi
4. GPi increases the inhibition of the thalamus
5. Motor cortex activity is suppressed

Subthalamic Nucleus

- Major excitatory nucleus
- Lésion → Hemiballismus

Substantia Nigra

- SNc: dopaminergic; degenerates in Parkinson's disease
- SNr: GABAergic; outputs to thalamus and superior colliculus

Nucleus Accumbens

- Integrates limbic and motor information
- Central to reward, motivation, and addiction

Clinical Disorders

Hypokinetic Disorders

Parkinson's disease

- Loss of SNc dopaminergic neurons
- Lewy bodies (αsynuclein)
- Bradykinesia, rigidity, resting tremor, postural instability

Updated diagnostics:

- αsynuclein seed amplification assays
- DaTscan

Updated treatments:

- Levodopa/carbidopa
- Dopamine agonists
- MAOB inhibitors
- COMT inhibitors
- Amantadine
- DBS (STN/GPi)
- Levodopa intestinal gel
- Emerging gene therapies

Secondary Parkinsonism: trauma, infection, toxins, medications, PSP, CBD, Lewy body dementia

Hyperkinetic Disorders

- Tremor
- Tics (Tourette syndrome)
- Dystonia
- Athetosis
- Chorea
- Myoclonus
- Ballismus (STN lesion)

Tourette syndrome (updated):

- Onset 3–9 years, male predominance
- Motor + vocal tics
- Treatment: CBIT, α2 agonists, antipsychotics, VMAT2 inhibitors, DBS

Review Questions

Q1. Which basal ganglia structure degenerates in Parkinson's disease?
Answer: Substantia nigra pars compacta.

Q2. Which pathway facilitates movement?
Answer: Direct pathway.

Q3. What is the major output nucleus of the basal ganglia?
Answer: Globus pallidus interna (Gipe).

Q4. Lesion of the subthalamic nucleus produces what movement disorder?
Answer: Hemiballismus.

Q5. Which neurotransmitter excites D1 neurons and inhibits D2 neurons?
Answer: Dopamine.

Q6. Which thalamic nuclei relay basal ganglia output to the cortex?
Answer: Ventral anterior (VA) and ventral lateral (VL).

Q7. What is the primary treatment for Parkinson's disease?
Answer: Levodopa (usually combined with carbidopa).

Clinical Vignettes

Vignette 1 — Difficulty Initiating Movement
A 68-year-old man presents with bradykinesia, rigidity, and resting tremor. MRI shows loss of midbrain pigmentation.
Affected structure: Substantia nigra pars compacta.

Vignette 2 — Violent Flinging Movements
A patient develops sudden, flinging movements of the right arm and leg after a stroke.
Damaged nucleus: Left subthalamic nucleus.

Vignette 3 — Tic Disorder in a Child
A 9-year-old boy has repetitive eye blinking and throat clearing relieved by performing the tic.
Diagnosis: Tourette syndrome.

Vignette 4 — Drug-Induced Parkinsonism
A patient on antipsychotics develops rigidity and bradykinesia.
Mechanism: Dopamine receptor blockade in the striatum.

Vignette 5 — Hyperkinetic Movements
A patient exhibits brief, irregular, unpredictable limb movements.
Term: Chorea.

Vignette 6 — Reward Pathway Activation
A young adult with stimulant addiction shows increased activity in a dopaminergic midbrain nucleus during drug anticipation.
Structure: Ventral tegmental area (VTA).

Vignette 7 — Levodopa Response
A patient with Parkinson's disease improves dramatically after starting levodopa. Why not give dopamine directly?
Explanation: Dopamine does not cross the blood–brain barrier.

References

- Kandel, E. R., Schwartz, J. H., Jessell, T. M., et al. *Principles of Neural Science.* McGraw-Hill.
- DeLong, M. R., & Wichmann, T. Basal ganglia circuits and movement disorders. *JAMA Neurology.*
- Lanciego, J. L., Luquin, N., & Obeso, J. A. Functional neuroanatomy of the basal ganglia. *Progress in Neurobiology.*
- Obeso, J. A., Stamelou, M., Goetz, C. G., et al. Past, present, and future of Parkinson's disease. *Lancet Neurology.*
- Albin, R. L., Young, A. B., & Penney, J. B. The functional anatomy of basal ganglia disorders. *Trends in Neurosciences.*

Chapter 32

Limbic System: Development, Components, and Hippocampal Architecture

Click here to view
Chapter Video: https://youtu.be/3XRIqayCZZ4

The limbic system comprises a complex network of interconnected cortical and subcortical structures that collectively govern emotion, affective behavior, motivation, learning, and memory. Its functional scope encompasses the full spectrum of human experience, ranging from reward, pleasure, and attachment to fear, anxiety, and memory consolidation. While mild memory decline may accompany normal aging, pathology within limbic structures can produce profound amnesia at any stage of life. A classic example is damage to the mammillary bodies, which leads to severe impairment of memory irrespective of age. The term *limbic*, meaning "bordering," was introduced by Pierre Paul Broca in 1878 to describe a group of structures forming a border along the medial aspect of the cerebral hemispheres, unified by both anatomical continuity and functional integration.

An understanding of the limbic system is best grounded in its embryological development. During the early three-vesicle stage, the neural tube differentiates into the prosencephalon, mesencephalon, and rhombencephalon. As development proceeds to the five-vesicle stage, rapid expansion of the telencephalic vesicles gives rise to the cerebral hemispheres and associated subcortical nuclei. This expansion causes the telencephalon to envelop the diencephalon. The medial wall of the telencephalon subsequently fuses with the lateral wall of the diencephalon, forming a bordering cortical region from which the principal limbic structures emerge, including the hippocampus, amygdala, septal nuclei, cingulate gyrus, mammillary bodies, ventral tegmental area, nucleus accumbens, and orbitofrontal cortex. These structures function collectively to regulate emotional expression, motivation, reward processing, and the formation of both short-term and long-term memories.

Within this system, the hippocampal formation occupies a central role in memory processing. In coronal section, it appears as a rolled structure along the floor of the inferior horn of the lateral ventricle, with its anterior expansion forming the pes hippocampi. Its characteristic seahorse-like configuration reflects inward cortical folding. Structurally, the hippocampal formation consists of the parahippocampal gyrus, entorhinal cortex, subiculum, and hippocampus proper, the latter comprising the Cornu Ammonis (CA1–CA4) fields. These regions are populated predominantly by pyramidal neurons, which serve as the principal output elements. Interposed between the hippocampus proper and subiculum lies the dentate gyrus, composed of granule cells that function as the primary input neurons of the hippocampal circuit.

The internal circuitry of the hippocampus is highly organized and follows a largely unidirectional flow, forming the classic trisynaptic circuit essential for memory formation. Multimodal sensory information first reaches the entorhinal cortex, which projects to the dentate gyrus via the perforant pathway. From the dentate gyrus, signals are transmitted to CA3 neurons through mossy fibers, and subsequently from CA3 to CA1 via the Schaffer collateral pathway. The CA1 region serves as the principal output zone, projecting to the subiculum, which in turn gives rise to efferent fibers that converge to form the fornix. This circuit underlies short-term memory formation, long-term memory consolidation, and spatial navigation.

The fornix constitutes the major output pathway of the hippocampus. Fibers emerging from the hippocampus form the alveus, which condenses into the fimbria and continues as the fornix. The paired crura of the fornix curve medially and anteriorly beneath the corpus callosum, uniting to form the body of the fornix. Transverse fibers between the crura create the forniceal commissure, enabling interhippocampal communication and facilitating the bilateral spread of epileptiform activity in temporal lobe seizures. At the level of the anterior commissure, each fornical column divides into precommissural and postcommissural components. The precommissural fibers project to the septal nuclei, preoptic area, and orbitofrontal cortex, whereas the postcommissural fibers terminate in the mammillary bodies. From the mammillary bodies, signals are relayed to the anterior thalamic nucleus via the mammillothalamic tract, and subsequently to the cingulate cortex, which projects back to the entorhinal cortex. This closed-loop circuit, known as the Papez circuit, forms the anatomical basis for learning, memory consolidation, and emotional processing.

The amygdala, located anterior to the hippocampus in the medial temporal lobe, is a key structure for emotional processing and autonomic regulation. It consists of multiple nuclear groups, of which the Corticomedial and basolateral groups are most significant. The Corticomedial group, receiving olfactory inputs, is relatively rudimentary in humans, whereas the basolateral group is highly developed and extensively interconnected with the prefrontal and cingulate cortices. Through these connections, the amygdala plays a dominant role in emotional learning, fear conditioning, and the modulation of memory. Its afferent inputs arise from the olfactory bulb, orbitofrontal cortex, cingulate gyrus, medial thalamus, and hypothalamus, while its efferent pathways include the stria terminalis and the ventral amygdalofugal pathway. These projections link emotional processing with autonomic and endocrine responses.

The functional importance of the amygdala is illustrated by Klüver–Bucy syndrome, a condition resulting from bilateral amygdala lesions. This syndrome is characterized by behavioral changes including docility, loss of fear and aggression, hypersexuality, hyperorality, and hyperphagia, reflecting profound disruption of emotional regulation.

The septal area, situated between the septum pellucidum and the anterior commissure, forms the anterior component of the limbic system. It is involved in emotional regulation, explicit memory, sexual behavior, and maternal responses. Lesions in this region lead to behavioral disinhibition and exaggerated emotional expression, highlighting its role in modulating affective states.

Although anatomically part of the hypothalamus, the mammillary bodies function as integral components of the limbic system. They receive afferent input from the hippocampus via the postcommissural fornix and project to the anterior thalamic nucleus. These connections are essential for memory formation and retrieval. Damage to the mammillary bodies, particularly in the context of thiamine deficiency, results in Wernicke–Korsakoff syndrome, characterized by acute encephalopathy followed by chronic memory impairment and confabulation.

The cingulate cortex serves as a major interface between emotion, cognition, and behavior. The anterior cingulate gyrus is closely connected with the orbitofrontal cortex, medial prefrontal cortex, and amygdala, and is involved in emotional processing, motivation, conflict monitoring, and the expression of affect. It also plays a role in socially relevant behaviors such as attachment and bonding. The posterior cingulate cortex contributes to spatial memory, environmental awareness, and higher-order processes such as empathy and perspective-taking. Lesions in this region impair navigation and reduce the ability to interpret emotional and social cues.

Integration of limbic processing with higher cortical functions occurs through the orbitofrontal and ventromedial prefrontal cortices. These regions receive both direct and indirect projections from the amygdala and are responsible for integrating emotional signals with decision making, impulse control, and social behavior. Damage to these areas results in disinhibition, impaired judgment, and socially inappropriate conduct.

The ventral tegmental area, located in the midbrain, represents the origin of the mesolimbic and mesocortical dopaminergic pathways. These projections extend to the nucleus accumbens, amygdala, hippocampus, and prefrontal cortex, forming the neural substrate of reward, motivation, reinforcement learning, and addiction. Activation of this system occurs both during the experience of reward and in anticipation of it, thereby driving goal-directed behavior.

Memory within the limbic network can be broadly classified into sensory, short-term (working), and long-term memory systems. Sensory memory retains transient impressions for a brief duration, while working memory holds information for seconds to minutes and requires active rehearsal. Long-term memory is established through processes such as synaptic consolidation and long-term potentiation. It is further divided into implicit (non-declarative) memory, which governs skills and habits and is largely mediated by the cerebellum and basal ganglia, and explicit (declarative) memory, which encompasses episodic and semantic memory and depends heavily on hippocampal and cortical networks. The amygdala enhances declarative memory by attaching emotional significance to experiences, thereby improving retention of emotionally salient events.

In summary, the limbic system represents an integrated network that links emotion, memory, and behavior through a series of highly organized anatomical and functional circuits. It's coordinated activity underlies not only fundamental survival behaviors but also the complex emotional and cognitive processes that define human experience.

Review Questions

Q1. Which pathway carries hippocampal output to the mammillary bodies?
Answer: Post commissural fornix.

Q2. Which hippocampal field is the primary output region?
Answer: CA1.

Q3. A lesion of the amygdala produces which classic syndrome?
Answer: Klüver–Bucy syndrome.

Q4. Which nucleus is the major input gateway to the hippocampus?
Answer: Entorhinal cortex.

Q5. Which limbic structure is essential for reward anticipation and addiction?
Answer: Ventral tegmental area (VTA).

Q6. Which structure degenerates in thiamine deficiency?
Answer: Mammillary bodies.

Q7. Which cingulate region is involved in spatial memory?
Answer: Posterior cingulate gyrus.

Clinical Vignettes

Vignette 1 — Emotional Flattening and Hypersexuality
A 52-year-old man becomes unusually docile, hypersexual, and overeats after bilateral temporal lobe injury.
Most likely damaged structure: Amygdala → Klüver–Bucy syndrome.

Vignette 2 — Severe Anterograde Amnesia
A malnourished patient presents with confusion, ataxia, and ophthalmoplegia. MRI shows mammillary body degeneration.
Diagnosis: Wernicke encephalopathy (progressing to Korsakoff syndrome).

Vignette 3 — Loss of Spatial Navigation
A patient struggles to navigate familiar environments and cannot orient objects in space.
Affected structure: Posterior cingulate gyrus.

Vignette 4 — RewardSeeking Behavior

A young adult with stimulant addiction shows heightened activation in a midbrain dopaminergic nucleus during drug anticipation.

Involved structure: Ventral tegmental area (VTA).

Vignette 5 — Impaired Emotional DecisionMaking

A patient with frontal lobe trauma displays impulsivity, poor judgment, and difficulty integrating emotional cues.

Damaged region: Ventromedial prefrontal cortex.

Vignette 6 — Memory Encoding Failure

A patient with hippocampal damage cannot form new long-term memories but retains procedural skills.

Preserved memory type: Implicit (procedural) memory.

References

1. Squire, L. R., Berg, D., Bloom, F. E., et al. *Fundamental Neuroscience.* Academic Press. Comprehensive coverage of hippocampal circuitry, amygdala function, and memory systems.
2. Bear, M. F., Connors, B. W., & Paradiso, M. A. *Neuroscience: Exploring the Brain.* Lippincott Williams & Wilkins. Clear explanations of limbic pathways, reward circuits, and emotional processing.
3. Nieuwenhuys, R., Voogd, J., & van Huijzen, C. *The Human Central Nervous System.* Springer. Detailed structural anatomy of limbic components, including hippocampus, fornix, and cingulate cortex.
4. Aggleton, J. P. *The Amygdala: A Functional Analysis.* Oxford University Press. — Authoritative source on amygdala subdivisions, connectivity, and behavioral roles.
5. Amaral, D. G., & Lavenex, P. *Hippocampal Neuroanatomy.* In: *The Hippocampus Book.* Oxford University Press. Goldstandard reference for hippocampal architecture, CA fields, and trisynaptic circuitry.

Chapter 33

Demyelinating Diseases of the CNS Classification, Pathophysiology, and Major Clinical Syndromes

Click here to view
Chapter Video: https://youtu.be/P4mclk9b4QE

Demyelinating diseases of the central nervous system constitute a group of disorders characterized by selective injury to myelin sheaths, with relative preservation of axons in the early stages. Because myelin is essential for rapid saltatory conduction along nerve fibers, its loss leads to impaired neural transmission, resulting in neurological deficits that may be transient or permanent depending on the degree of inflammation, the capacity for remyelination, and the extent of secondary axonal damage. These disorders may arise from primary processes intrinsic to the central nervous system or occur secondary to systemic, metabolic, infectious, or toxic insults. A clear understanding of this classification provides the foundation for accurate diagnosis and appropriate management.

Primary demyelinating disorders are those in which myelin is directly targeted by immune-mediated or idiopathic mechanisms. Among these, autoimmune and inflammatory conditions predominate. **Multiple sclerosis** represents the prototypical disorder in this category, accompanied by other important entities such as Neuromyelitis optica spectrum disorder, MOG antibody–associated disease, Acute disseminated encephalomyelitis, and Acute transverse myelitis. In addition, certain idiopathic forms, including progressive solitary sclerosis and tumefactive demyelination, present diagnostic challenges due to their atypical features and resemblance to neoplastic processes.

Secondary demyelinating disorders arise from external or systemic factors that indirectly damage myelin. Infectious causes include HIVassociated demyelination and Progressive multifocal leukoencephalopathy, the latter resulting from reactivation of the JC virus in immunocompromised individuals. Metabolic and nutritional deficiencies, particularly vitamin B12 deficiency leading to subacute combined degeneration, copper deficiency, and severe hypoxia, are also well-recognized causes. Toxic insults such as chemotherapy, especially methotrexate, radiation exposure, and environmental toxins may similarly disrupt myelin integrity. In addition, systemic autoimmune conditions such as lupus cerebritis and Sjögren-related central nervous system involvement may produce secondary demyelination through immune-mediated mechanisms.

Among all demyelinating diseases, multiple sclerosis remains the most extensively studied and clinically significant. It is a chronic, immune-mediated disorder characterized by lesions disseminated in both time and space, reflecting episodic inflammatory activity affecting different regions of the central nervous system at different times. It is the most common disabling neurological disease of young adults, with peak onset between 20 and 40 years of age and a marked female predominance. Its geographic distribution shows higher prevalence in temperate regions, a pattern partly attributed to environmental factors such as vitamin D deficiency.

The **etiology of multiple sclerosis** is multifactorial, involving an interplay between genetic susceptibility, environmental exposures, and immune dysregulation. Genetic factors include associations with specific HLA haplotypes, while environmental contributors include prior infection with Epstein–Barr virus, reduced sunlight exposure, and smoking. At the immunological level, autoreactive T lymphocytes, B cells, and other immune effectors infiltrate the central nervous system, initiating an inflammatory cascade that targets myelin.

The **pathological hallmark of multiple sclerosis** is immune-mediated demyelination. Activated $CD4^+$ and $CD8^+$ T cells, along with B cells and macrophages, cross the blood–brain barrier and attack myelin sheaths. Microglial activation further amplifies this process. Although oligodendrocytes may initially survive, allowing partial remyelination during remission, repeated inflammatory episodes eventually lead to gliosis and the formation of sclerotic plaques. In chronic stages, axonal loss becomes prominent and contributes to irreversible neurological disability.

A **defining feature of multiple sclerosis** is the distribution of lesions in both time and space. Lesions may occur in the optic nerves, brainstem, cerebellum, spinal cord, and periventricular white matter, producing a wide spectrum of clinical manifestations. Patients commonly present with optic neuritis, characterized by painful visual loss, as well as diplopia due to internuclear ophthalmoplegia, sensory disturbances, motor weakness, ataxia, and bladder dysfunction. The clinical course is often relapsing and remitting, although some individuals eventually develop a progressive form with steady neurological decline.

Diagnosis of multiple sclerosis is primarily clinical but is strongly supported by neuroimaging and laboratory findings. Magnetic resonance imaging reveals characteristic lesions in periventricular, juxtacortical, infratentorial, and spinal cord regions, with gadolinium enhancement indicating active inflammation. Cerebrospinal fluid analysis frequently demonstrates oligoclonal bands and an elevated IgG index, reflecting intrathecal immunoglobulin synthesis. Evoked potential studies provide additional evidence by demonstrating slowed conduction consistent with demyelination.

In contrast to the multifocal nature of multiple sclerosis, **acute transverse myelitis** represents a focal inflammatory demyelinating disorder of the spinal cord. Acute transverse myelitis typically presents with a rapid onset of bilateral motor weakness, a well-defined sensory level, and autonomic dysfunction affecting bowel and bladder control. The condition may develop over hours to days and can occur at any age without a clear demographic predilection. While a substantial proportion of cases are idiopathic, others are associated with autoimmune diseases, including multiple sclerosis, neuromyelitis optica spectrum disorder, and MOG antibody–associated disease.

The diagnosis of acute transverse myelitis relies on imaging and cerebrospinal fluid analysis. Magnetic resonance imaging reveals focal inflammation within the spinal cord, while cerebrospinal fluid studies often show pleocytosis and elevated protein levels. It is essential to exclude compressive lesions, such as tumors or epidural abscesses, which may present with similar clinical features but require different management. The prognosis of acute transverse myelitis is variable, with some patients achieving complete recovery and others developing persistent neurological deficits.

In summary, demyelinating diseases of the central nervous system represent a diverse group of disorders unified by the common mechanism of myelin injury. They may be primary, arising from intrinsic immune-mediated or idiopathic processes, or secondary to systemic, infectious, metabolic, or toxic causes. Among these, multiple sclerosis remains the most important prototype, illustrating the principles of immune-mediated demyelination, lesion dissemination, and clinical variability. Acute transverse myelitis exemplifies a focal inflammatory process affecting the spinal cord. Together, these conditions highlight the critical role of myelin in maintaining normal neurological function and underscore the importance of early recognition and intervention in preventing long-term disability.

Consolidated Summary Sheet

Demyelinating diseases are disorders in which myelin sheaths of the CNS are damaged, leading to impaired conduction, neurological deficits, and, depending on the cause, either relapsing or progressive disability. They may be primary (immune-mediated or idiopathic) or secondary (due to systemic or environmental insults).

Classification of Demyelinating Disorders

E. **Primary Demyelinating Disorders**

Intrinsic immune-mediated or idiopathic processes targeting CNS myelin.

1. Autoimmune / Inflammatory
    - Multiple sclerosis (MS)
    - Neuromyelitis optica spectrum disorder (NMOSD)
    - MOGantibody–associated disease (MOGAD)
    - Acute disseminated encephalomyelitis (ADEM)
    - Acute transverse myelitis (ATM)
2. Idiopathic
    - Progressive solitary sclerosis
    - Tumefactive demyelination

F. **Secondary Demyelinating Disorders**

Occur due to external or systemic insults.

1. Infectious
    - HIVassociated demyelination
    - Progressive multifocal leukoencephalopathy (PML) — JC virus
    - Post-infectious demyelination
2. Metabolic / Nutritional
    - Vitamin B12 deficiency (subacute combined degeneration)
    - Copper deficiency
    - Severe hypoxia

3. Toxic
   - Chemotherapy (e.g., methotrexate)
   - Radiation-induced demyelination
   - Environmental toxins

4. Systemic Autoimmune
   - Lupus cerebritis
   - Sjögren-related demyelination

Review Questions

Q1. What is the hallmark pathological feature of MS?
Answer: Patchy demyelination with relative axonal sparing.

Q2. What two criteria define MS lesions?
Answer: Dissemination in time and space.

Q3. Which antibody is associated with neuromyelitis optica spectrum disorder (NMOSD)?
Answer: Anti-AQP4 (aquaporin4) antibodies.

Q4. What CSF finding supports a diagnosis of MS?
Answer: Oligoclonal IgG bands.

Q5. What is the most common initial symptom of MS?
Answer: Optic neuritis.

Q6. What is the most common cause of acute transverse myelitis?
Answer: Idiopathic (60%).

Q7. Which vitamin deficiency causes secondary demyelination of the dorsal columns?
Answer: Vitamin B12 deficiency.

Clinical Vignettes

Vignette 1 MS
A 28yearold woman presents with painful vision loss in one eye and an MRI showing periventricular lesions. CSF reveals oligoclonal bands.
Diagnosis: Multiple sclerosis.

Vignette 2 Acute Transverse Myelitis
A 35yearold develops rapidly progressive bilateral leg weakness and urinary retention. MRI shows focal spinal cord inflammation.
Diagnosis: Acute transverse myelitis.

Vignette 3 Secondary Demyelination
A patient with chronic alcoholism presents with gait ataxia and loss of vibration sense. Labs show low vitamin B12.
Diagnosis: Subacute combined degeneration.

Vignette 4 NMOSD
A patient presents with severe optic neuritis and longitudinally extensive transverse myelitis. Serum AQP4 antibodies are positive.
Diagnosis: Neuromyelitis optica spectrum disorder.

Vignette 5 MOGAD
A child develops optic neuritis and ADEM-like lesions after a viral illness. Serum MOG antibodies are positive.
Diagnosis: MOGassociated demyelinating disease.

References

1. Squire, L. R., Berg, D., Bloom, F. E., et al. *Fundamental Neuroscience.* Academic Press. Comprehensive coverage of hippocampal circuitry, amygdala function, and memory systems.
2. Bear, M. F., Connors, B. W., & Paradiso, M. A. *Neuroscience: Exploring the Brain.* Lippincott Williams & Wilkins. Clear explanations of limbic pathways, reward circuits, and emotional processing.

Chapter 34

Degenerative Disorders of Central Nervous System: Classification, Neurobiology, and Major Clinical Syndromes

Click here to view
Chapter Video: https://youtu.be/-pi1IHrMyuc

Degenerative disorders of the central nervous system represent a group of chronic, progressive conditions characterized by selective or widespread neuronal loss, accumulation of abnormal proteins, synaptic dysfunction, and eventual structural atrophy. These disorders evolve over years to decades and reflect fundamental disturbances in neuronal maintenance, protein homeostasis, and network integrity. Broadly, they may be classified as primary degenerative disorders, in which neuronal loss arises intrinsically without an identifiable external cause, or secondary degenerative disorders, in which neuronal injury is triggered by systemic, metabolic, toxic, or infectious factors. This distinction is clinically important, as secondary causes may be preventable or reversible if recognized early.

Secondary degeneration occurs in response to identifiable insults such as toxic exposures, metabolic derangements, chronic alcohol use, nutritional deficiencies, or infections. Heavy metals, organic solvents, and radiation may directly damage neurons, while metabolic conditions such as hepatic failure or Wilson's disease produce neurotoxicity through the accumulation of toxic metabolites. Chronic alcohol consumption and thiamine deficiency may lead to Wernicke–Korsakoff syndrome, a condition marked by profound memory impairment. Infectious etiologies, including HIV and neurosyphilis, can also result in progressive neuronal loss. Importantly, early identification and treatment of these underlying causes may halt or even reverse neurological decline.

In contrast, **primary degenerative disorders** arise from intrinsic neuronal dysfunction and are further divided into diffuse (global) and selective (system-based) forms. Diffuse degenerative disorders involve widespread cortical and subcortical regions and commonly present as dementia syndromes. The major entities in this category include Alzheimer's disease, Lewy body dementia, Frontotemporal dementia, and vascular dementia, which often coexist with other pathologies. Selective degenerative disorders, on the other hand, affect specific neuronal systems or circuits, such as the dopaminergic system in Parkinson's disease, the striatal neurons in Huntington's disease, or upper and lower motor neurons in Amyotrophic lateral sclerosis.

Dementia, a central clinical manifestation of many diffuse degenerative disorders, is best understood as a syndrome rather than a single disease entity. It is characterized by progressive decline in memory, impairment of executive function, behavioral and personality changes, and eventual loss of functional independence. The pattern of early symptoms often reflects the underlying pathology. For example, Alzheimer's disease typically presents with early short-term memory impairment, Lewy body dementia is notable for fluctuating cognition and visual hallucinations, and frontotemporal dementia often begins with personality changes or language disturbances.

Among these conditions, Alzheimer's disease is the most common cause of dementia worldwide. It is a slowly progressive neurodegenerative disorder with a prolonged preclinical phase during which pathological changes may begin years before the onset of symptoms. Its etiology is multifactorial, involving genetic predisposition, particularly the APOE ε4 allele, age-related metabolic changes, neuroinflammation, and impaired clearance of abnormal proteins.

The **pathophysiology of Alzheimer's** disease is defined by two major molecular abnormalities. The first involves dysfunction of the amyloid pathway, in which abnormal processing of the amyloid precursor protein leads to the accumulation of β-amyloid peptides, particularly Aβ42. These peptides aggregate to form extracellular amyloid plaques, which disrupt synaptic function, trigger neuroinflammation, and impair neurotransmission. The second hallmark is tau pathology, in which hyperphosphorylation of the microtubule-associated protein tau leads to destabilization of microtubules and formation of intracellular neurofibrillary tangles. These tangles interfere with axonal transport and correlate strongly with cognitive decline.

As the disease progresses, neuronal atrophy becomes evident, initially affecting the hippocampus and entorhinal cortex, which explains the early impairment of memory. With advancing disease, degeneration extends to the temporal, parietal, and frontal lobes, ultimately resulting in global cortical atrophy. Clinically, Alzheimer's disease progresses through stages, beginning with mild memory impairment and subtle cognitive deficits, advancing to confusion, disorientation, and behavioral changes, and culminating in severe global cognitive decline with loss of motor function and complete dependency.

Lewy body dementia represents another major cause of degenerative cognitive decline and is classified as a Synucleinopathy. It is characterized by fluctuating cognition, recurrent visual hallucinations, and Parkinsonian motor features. The underlying pathology involves the accumulation of α-synuclein within neurons, forming intracytoplasmic inclusions known as Lewy bodies. These are distributed across the cortex, midbrain, hypothalamus, and substantia nigra. Neurochemically, there is a marked deficiency of acetylcholine, contributing to cognitive impairment, along with progressive dopaminergic loss, which accounts for motor symptoms. Imaging may reveal cortical atrophy and involvement of subcortical structures, although definitive diagnosis remains clinical and is confirmed histopathologically.

Frontotemporal dementia differs from Alzheimer's disease in both its age of onset and clinical presentation. Typically affecting individuals between 40 and 60 years of age, it primarily involves degeneration of the frontal and temporal lobes. The behavioral variant is characterized by profound personality changes, disinhibition, loss of empathy, and compulsive behaviors. Language variants include progressive non-fluent aphasia, marked by effortful and halting speech, and semantic dementia, in which patients lose the meaning of words and the ability to recognize objects despite fluent speech. Because it affects individuals in their most productive years, frontotemporal dementia carries significant social and occupational consequences.

Selective degenerative disorders, although discussed in detail elsewhere, illustrate the principle of system-specific neuronal vulnerability. Parkinson's disease results from degeneration of dopaminergic neurons in the substantia nigra, leading to hypokinetic motor symptoms. Huntington's disease is a genetic disorder characterized by CAG repeat expansion, resulting in progressive degeneration of the caudate nucleus and hyperkinetic movements. Amyotrophic lateral sclerosis involves degeneration of both upper and lower motor neurons, leading to progressive weakness and eventual respiratory failure.

In summary, degenerative disorders of the central nervous system are defined by progressive neuronal loss, abnormal protein aggregation, and disruption of neural networks. They may be primary, arising from intrinsic neurodegenerative processes, or secondary to systemic or environmental factors. Diffuse forms typically present with dementia, while selective forms affect specific motor or cognitive systems. Among these, Alzheimer's disease, Lewy body dementia, and frontotemporal dementia represent the major causes of cortical degeneration, each with distinct pathological mechanisms and clinical profiles. Understanding these disorders provides critical insight into the relationship between brain structure, molecular pathology, and clinical function.

Consolidated Summary Sheet

Degenerative disorders of the CNS are chronic, progressive conditions characterized by selective or diffuse neuronal loss, abnormal protein accumulation, synaptic dysfunction, and eventual structural atrophy. They may be primary (intrinsic neuronal degeneration) or secondary (due to external/systemic causes).

Classification of Degenerative Disorders

A. **Secondary Degeneration**

Occurs due to identifiable causes:

- Toxic exposures (heavy metals, solvents, radiation)
- Metabolic disorders
- Chronic alcohol use
- Nutritional deficiencies (e.g., thiamine deficiency)
- Infections (HIV, neurosyphilis)

Potentially reversible if the underlying cause is treated early.

B. **Primary Degeneration**

1. **Diffuse (Global) Degeneration**

   Affects widespread cortical and subcortical regions.

   Major disorders:

   - Alzheimer's disease (AD)
   - Lewy body dementia (LBD)
   - Frontotemporal dementia (FTD)
   - Vascular dementia

2. **Selective/System-Based Degeneration**
   Affects specific neuronal circuits.
   Major disorders:
   - Parkinson's disease
   - Huntington's disease
   - Motor neuron disease (ALS)

Review Questions

Q1. What are the two major pathological hallmarks of Alzheimer's disease?
Answer: Amyloid plaques and neurofibrillary tangles.

Q2. Which protein accumulates in Lewy body dementia?
Answer: αsynuclein.

Q3. Which dementia often presents with early hallucinations and fluctuating cognition?
Answer: Lewy body dementia.

Q4. Which brain region is affected earliest in Alzheimer's disease?
Answer: Hippocampus.

Q5. What is the typical age range for frontotemporal dementia onset?
Answer: 40–60 years.

Q6. Which degenerative disorder is associated with progressive non-fluent aphasia?
Answer: Frontotemporal dementia.

Q7. What neurotransmitter is markedly reduced in Lewy body dementia?
Answer: Acetylcholine.

Clinical Vignettes

Vignette 1 — Alzheimer's Disease

A 72-year-old presents with progressive short-term memory loss and difficulty understanding language. MRI shows hippocampal atrophy.
Diagnosis: Alzheimer's disease.

Vignette 2 — Lewy Body Dementia
A 68-year-old reports vivid visual hallucinations and fluctuating alertness. Later develops bradykinesia and rigidity.
Diagnosis: Lewy body dementia.

Vignette 3 — Frontotemporal Dementia
A 52-year-old becomes socially inappropriate, impulsive, and emotionally indifferent. Speech remains intact.
Diagnosis: Behavioral variant FTD.

Vignette 4 — Semantic Dementia
A patient speaks fluently but cannot name common objects or understand word meanings.
Diagnosis: Semantic variant FTD.

Vignette 5 — Progressive Non-Fluent Aphasia
A patient has effortful, halting speech with intact comprehension.
Diagnosis: Non-fluent variant FTD.

References

1. Neuroanatomy Through Clinical Cases
   Blumenfeld H. *Neuroanatomy Through Clinical Cases*. 3rd ed. Sinauer Associates.
2. Principles of Neural Science
   Kandel ER, et al. *Principles of Neural Science*. 6th ed. McGraw-Hill.
3. Bear, M. F., Connors, B. W., & Paradiso, M. A. *Neuroscience: Exploring the Brain*. Lippincott Williams & Wilkins.

Note to Students

Companion titles, available as video-embedded e books and in print formats:

- *Clinical Embryology* - The principles of human development with clinical correlations.
- *Essentials of Medical Genetics* - A concise reference outlining fundamental genetic concepts and their medical applications.

These volumes are intended to provide an integrated foundation across related disciplines.

Author's Note

Neuroscience is a field that is evolving rapidly, yet its foundational principles remain remarkably stable. As an educator and academic author, I have always believed that clarity, conceptual integration, and clinical relevance are the pillars of effective learning. This E-Book and its multimedia content reflect the underlying philosophy.

The manuscript has evolved from my teaching experience in neuroanatomy, developmental biology, and genetics, as well as my work in clinical cytogenetics. Over time, I have observed that students learn most effectively when complex concepts are presented in a structured, narrative format, one that connects pathways to behavior, anatomy to function, and clinical signs to their underlying mechanisms.

This book, with its streamlined, integrated, and student-friendly content, will hopefully complement the comprehensive textbooks on this subject quite substantially. It is written with the learner in mind: concise where it must be, detailed where it matters, and always anchored in the logic of neuroanatomy.

www.ingramcontent.com/pod-product-compliance
Lightning Source LLC
LaVergne TN
LVHW022208200926
848481LV00006B/1890